Why Can't We Have a Baby?

Why Can't We Have a Baby?

AN AUTHORITY LOOKS
AT THE
CAUSES AND CURES OF
CHILDLESSNESS

BY ALBERT DECKER, M.D.
AND SUZANNE LOEBL

THE DIAL PRESS   NEW YORK

Published by
The Dial Press
1 Dag Hammarskjold Plaza
New York, New York 10017

Manufactured in the United States of America

First printing

Library of Congress Cataloging in Publication Data

Decker, Albert.
Why can't we have a baby?

Includes index.
1. Sterility.   I. Loebl, Suzanne, joint
author.   II. Title.
RC889.D4   618.1'78   78–6996
ISBN 0–8037–9567–X

For all would-be parents

ACKNOWLEDGMENTS

Much of the material in this book was derived from the clinical experience of the senior author, who has spent more than fifty years helping couples overcome their infertility problems.

To list all the books and articles used as additional background material would be an impossible task. Sources include original scientific writings, public lectures, textbooks, and magazine articles. We thank all those whose work enabled us to write this book.

We also want to thank the many patients kind enough to share their experiences with us, thereby making the task of those who will have to travel the same path a little easier.

Thanks is also due to the many busy investigators and professionals interviewed in the course of our research. Their first-hand accounts of important developments were of great value. Thanks to: Richard D. Amelar, Miriam Biddelman, Wayne H. Decker, Karl Eric Johanson, Masood A. Katamee, Georgeanna S. Jones, Ernest Lieber, Landrum B. Shettles, Sidney Shulman, and Don M. Sloan. Albert Rosenfeld, Lynn Yates, and David R. Zimmerman also deserve thanks for their suggestions and special help. Though their help cannot be overestimated, we alone are responsible for any possible errors or misinterpretations.

Last but not least, we want to thank our families for being patient with us during the time this book was conceived and written.

CONTENTS

ONE

INTRODUCTION

1

FIRST VISIT

And when Rachel saw that she bore Jacob no children, Rachel envied her sister; and she said unto Jacob: "Give me children or else I die."

Genesis 30:1

PEOPLE HAVE DIFFERENT IDEAS ABOUT THEIR FERTILITY. SOME WOMEN expect to become pregnant "right away"; others are very surprised when they do conceive after a few months. Some men fear sterility and its fancied connection with impotence; others speculate about their limitless power to impregnate. Nevertheless, in spite of these fantasies, when a particular couple realizes that they have, or may have, a fertility problem, they are terribly shocked. At the bottom of our hearts we all expect to "beget" children without much trouble. Even to the nonreligious the word "barren" sounds almost like a curse.

Yet the problem is a rather common one. Fifteen percent of all couples, or one couple in eight, have trouble conceiving.

In bygone days a couple who wondered why they did not conceive might have intensified their prayers, tried some kind of folk remedy, or visited a special shrine. Today most couples will decide sooner or later to visit a physician.

The time when you should seek help depends on the age of the wife. A woman in her early twenties has many years during which she can bear children. Even though her fertility will be at its maximum at about age twenty-five, she can afford to wait twelve to eighteen months before consulting a physician if she thinks she may have a problem.

A physician should be consulted sooner when the wife is from twenty-six to thirty-two years old. Finally, women beyond the age of thirty-two, who are approaching the end of their reproductive years, should visit a physician promptly if pregnancy does not occur within six months.

The decision to consult a physician is not an easy one. It has been said that there are two subjects about which people tell more lies than any other: money and sex. If you go to see a physician about your infertility problem, he or she will obviously include a discussion of your sex life.

The subject was taboo for our Victorian forebears, and until recently even doctors were most reluctant to discuss sex with their patients. Today we are more candid about these matters. Yet sexual liberation has brought with it new pressures. The couple may wonder whether their sex life is "good" enough.

The couple also may believe that only one of them will be responsible for their failure to have children. (In reality, infertility often results from a combination of male and female factors.) They wonder what this knowledge will do to their relationship. The man knows that his fertility will be measured and counted in no uncertain terms, and the woman probably dreads the many gynecological examinations that may be in store for her.

It cannot be emphasized too often that a person's actual fertility rating has nothing to do with his or her capacity to be an excellent, passionate lover. Infertility is a medical problem, and should be so considered. Patients who are struggling to overcome their infertility today are in a much better position than were those similarly affected as little as ten years ago.

Since infertility is a subject fraught with emotion, it is most important that the couple like the physician with whom they will entrust one of the most crucial issues of their lives.

Finding a good doctor is never an easy matter, and since

infertility has been neglected for a very long time, there are not too many physicians who specialize in this area. In important medical matters it may also be desirable to consult a second physician, not because one does not trust one's regular physician but because it is reassuring to have a second opinion. The wife's gynecologist or the regular family physician are obviously the first resources to be consulted. These doctors themselves may wish to call in a consultant, and may be entirely competent to recommend another specialist.

A couple may also decide that they wish to choose their own consultant, either because they feel that a request for a consultation may indicate a lack of confidence in their primary care physician or because they wish an entirely independent opinion. Recommendations from friends are a good way of finding a doctor. In addition, every county medical society maintains a list of specialists, and the American Fertility Society (1608 13th Avenue South # 101, Birmingham, Alabama, 35205; 205–933–7222) maintains a complete list of infertility specialists practicing in the United States. There are also clinics and institutions that specialize in infertility research. An infertility clinic or medical group is often more desirable than a physician in individual practice because such an institution is staffed by a group of doctors, each one particularly knowledgeable in one aspect of the field.

When you have identified the physician you wish to consult, it is entirely appropriate to ask over the telephone about fees, experience, what hospital he or she is associated with, and other important questions. Many of these will be answered by the office nurse or receptionist. If you live in a large city, you may be fortunate in uncovering the names of several physicians who specialize in infertility. In that case you may be able to make an intelligent judgment on the basis of your telephone interview.

Once you have settled on a particular individual, it is a good idea to give the physician a chance to solve the problem. Patients who readily change doctors usually do worse than those who give themselves and their physician a chance.

The Initial Visit

People judge each other very quickly, and the basis of a good doctor-patient relationship is often cemented during the initial visit.

Both the husband and the wife should go on this first visit. No matter whether both or only one eventually turn out to be responsible for the difficulties disclosed, both partners must become seriously involved.

First impressions are very important, and most physicians have learned how to judge a couple quickly. Are they loving? Embarrassed? Mad at each other? Supportive? Do they wish a child simply and desperately to save a crumbling marriage, or is their bond strong enough to adjust to and accept the disappointment of being childless. (At the New York Fertility Research Foundation a patient is not accepted if the child is wanted only to buttress a crumbling marriage.)

Are they both sincere in their quest for parenthood? Is the husband as earnestly involved as the wife, and will he cooperate completely? Does the wife want pregnancy to satisfy a desire on the part of the husband or either set of relatives? Does the woman consciously or unconsciously fear, or not desire, pregnancy?

It is also especially important to determine whether the wife's physical condition is capable of withstanding the strain of pregnancy and childbearing.

Finally, the physician will have to decide whether the patients are motivated enough to follow the sometimes complex instructions and procedures involved in overcoming infertility.

The cure of infertility, like that of most other medical conditions, is dependent upon three variables:

1—The type and severity of the problem.
2—The medical resources available to the patients—including the skill of the physician.

3—The motivation and determination of the patients.

While the physician evaluates the new patients, the patients also will be evaluating the physician. Will their problem be taken seriously? Will their story be listened to, even if it is told hesitantly and in clumsy words? Is the physician versed in the subject matter? Will matters be explained in "plain English" or will communication be restricted to medical jargon? Will the patients mean more to the doctor than two ovaries, one uterus, and two testicles?

Infertility can be caused by a great variety of factors, or combinations of factors, most of which will be discussed in the pages of this book. Sometimes the cause is simple; often it is complex. Sometimes the malfunction is traced to the husband, sometimes to the wife. Often it is a combination of both.

Table I (pp.8–9) lists common causes of infertility for both men and women.

Although much progress has been made in infertility research over the last decades, not every couple—even if they have the best medical advice and are highly motivated—can expect to become parents. But practically everyone should be able to find out why they failed to conceive. And while it may at first be difficult to learn that a particular infertility problem cannot be remedied, it is far better, in the long run, to adjust to such a situation than to keep hoping indefinitely.

The physician's first task usually is to take a careful medical history. How old is the husband, the wife? How long have they been married? How long have they been trying to have a baby? How often do they have intercourse? What are their occupations? Has either had children by other partners? Was there an abortion, spontaneous or induced? How regularly does the wife menstruate? How old was she when she first menstruated? Are her periods painful? Did she have rubella? Did he

TABLE I
Common Causes of Infertility

Female	Male

GENERAL

Female	Male
Overweight	*Overweight*
Underweight	*Underweight*
Anemia	*Excess alcohol*
	Excess smoking

DEVELOPMENTAL

Female	Male
Uterine malformations	*Undescended testicles*
Underdeveloped ovaries	*Varicocele*
Incompetent cervix	*Underdeveloped testicles*
	Poor sperm count

ENDOCRINE

Female	Male
Pituitary failure	*Pituitary failure*
Thyroid defects	*Thyroid disease*
Ovarian failure	*Adrenal overdevelopment*
(Stein-Leventhal Disease)	*Poor sperm count*
Adrenal overdevelopment	
Hostile mucus	

GENITAL DISEASE

Female	Male
Endometriosis	*Venereal disease*

have mumps as an adult? Did either of them have surgery, and if so when, and of what kind?

Many a potential problem can be pinpointed by such questions. An irregular menstrual cycle may indicate a problem with ovulation. Very painful periods may indicate endometriosis. Very infrequent intercourse may reduce the chances of con-

TABLE I *(cont'd)*
Common Causes of Infertility

Female	Male

GENITAL DISEASE *(cont'd)*

Female	Male
Cervical polyps	*Injury to testes*
Uterine polyps	*Hydrocele*
Uterine fibroids	*Orchitis*
Infections: venereal, tuberculosis,	*Prostatitis*
monilia, mycoplasm, cervicitis,	
tubal infections	

GENETIC DISEASE

Female	Male
Turner's Syndrome	*Klinefelter Syndrome*

PSYCHOLOGICAL FACTORS

Female	Male
Vaginismus	*Impotence*
Fear	*Ejaculation, premature*
	ejaculation, retardate
	ejaculation, retrograde

Male-Female Factors

Marital maladjustment
Misunderstanding of fertile days
Immunological incompatibility
(antibodies to sperm)

ception. Only a thorough examination and specialized tests will confirm or rule out these suspicions.

Patients who consult a physician about a medical problem of any kind do well to tell the truth. But any physician who has been in practice for some time knows that this is not always possible, at least not right away.

Husbands and wives do have secrets from one another. The wife may want to hide an abortion or even a previous pregnancy. People lie about their ages, venereal disease, their sexual mores, the "hell they raised in their youth," and many other things that may or may not have a bearing on the problem of their infertility.

Sometimes the medical problem that patients announce when they make their initial appointment is only the official admission ticket. It will take time, and confidence in the doctor, to allow the true cause of their concern to be ferreted out. During the initial interview the doctor must be very careful to "open the door" so that such problems can eventually be discussed.

In this first visit the physician may wish to explain and indoctrinate the couple as to the routine required to determine the cause for failure. They may be supplied with printed material and instructions concerning scheduling and preparation for the necessary tests.

The survey usually starts with a determination of the fertility status of the husband, which can be established by two simple tests (sperm count and postcoital test). If these are satisfactory, the husband can be considered normally fertile.

The physician also should inform both husband and wife, at the outset, that an infertility investigation may take months to complete. Treatment undertaken to correct a particular problem often takes still longer. Even after the problem has been diagnosed and treatment is available, it often takes years before you will hold a child in your arms. Do not become discouraged. The chances of an infertile couple conceiving increase every year. Though exact figures are hard to come by, it is estimated that 67 percent of every 100 couples who have an infertility problem will eventually produce a healthy baby with some medical help.

On the other hand, it often happens that a patient who seeks help is found to be pregnant on her first or second visit to the infertility specialist, before she had a chance to turn to the prescribed therapy.

After the joint interview the patients will be examined individually. But before we delve into a detailed description of specific tests and treatments, let us look at the emotions that the specter of infertility arouses in those who have to deal with this particular medical problem.

2

WHY US?

Once again my body tells me a
Child to bear is not my fate
The days fly past in their pain
Why in the past did I hesitate
Wanting so terribly needing to know
My love will find a place
Why is there no justice, Why such a waste?

—Infertility patient

EVERY TUESDAY, AT 5:30 SHARP, FIVE YOUNG WOMEN ASSEMBLE AT THE New York Fertility Research Foundation in New York. Although they come from different backgrounds and different races they are closely united because they all are attempting to become pregnant.

The healing power of a group of patients who share a common problem was discovered almost fifty years ago by Dr. Joseph Pratt of Boston, who treated a group of patients suffering from tuberculosis. The preferred treatment at the time was to send patients to fancy, expensive sanatoria in Colorado or the Adirondacks, which not everybody could afford. Dr. Pratt assembled some of those left behind in the slums of Boston and organized his Classes for the Treatment of Tuberculosis in the Homes of the Poor. The topic to be discussed was how to make the most of the meager fresh-air resources of the city.

To everybody's surprise these patients did as well as, or better than, those who went to the mountains. Since the Boston air even then was not all that good, it was concluded that the patients profited from the healing power of what came to be called "a common bond in a common disease." This was the beginning of group therapy.

Dr. Pratt's patients had a strictly physiological disease, whereas group therapy has been mostly used for patients suffering from various psychological and social disorders. But today there is increased recognition that all patients who share any kind of serious problem profit from sharing their fears and frustrations with others who are in the same situation. Infertility is no exception.

The women who assemble on Tuesdays in New York are very fortunate because their group leader, Miriam Biddelman, is one of the very few psychiatric social workers in America who decided to specialize in working with infertility patients.

These group members are at various stages of their battle with infertility. Some have just begun to face the fact that they may never bear their own children. Others have been coming to the group for nearly two years, all the while undergoing various therapeutic procedures, hoping, praying, crying, raging, and eventually coping.

There are a lot of tears. Some patients cry when they first come to the group. They always knew that they wanted children and planned their lives expecting to raise a family. Other women join the group in a more detached manner because they had never been convinced that they wanted children in the first place. Then, after they tried and failed, they started to suspect that they really wanted children all along.

Couples who have an infertility problem are bound to go through a severe emotional crisis. The possibility of remaining childless assaults a person's deep needs and sense of self. It necessitates a re-evaluation of one's lifestyle. Those involved must not only weather questions from family and friends, but also adjust their self-image.

For a while both the husband and the wife will feel emotionally and physically diminished because their ability to procreate is in doubt. Such reactions are entirely normal. It can almost be said that not feeling a deep sense of anxiety and loss is abnormal.

Most patients find Miriam Biddelman's group very supportive. Indeed one member reported that when she missed a period and believed herself to be pregnant—it turned out to be false hope—her first thought was that she would no longer be entitled to come to the group.

One may wonder why these groups usually are all female, even though infertility clearly is a major problem for both partners in a marriage. The reason, according to Miriam Biddelman, is that contemporary society does not yet permit men to express themselves emotionally as freely as women. To cry is still considered unmanly. (Patients who wish to be treated with their husband as a couple can opt for individual psychotherapy.)

But, even though they are not there in person, the men figure prominently in the discussion of "Miriam's group." Some men are reluctant to have their sperm counted. (If there is absolute refusal, the problem can be circumvented by using a postcoital test as a sperm count.) An infertility problem often causes a breakdown in communications between husband and wife. Again, this difficulty can frequently be traced to the husband's reluctance to allow his feelings of anxiety and disappointment to rise to the surface.

Many women feel that their husbands fail to give them sufficient emotional support.

Sex, which only recently emerged from centuries of prudery and inhibition, now becomes a chore. This is not surprising, since for infertility patients it often becomes a command performance during the forty-eight or so hours when a woman is fertile. Shared sexual pleasure can be totally eliminated when a sample must be obtained routinely by masturbation so that it can be used for artificial insemination.

One woman, who reported that both she and her husband faced their infertility problem without their marriage undergoing a major crisis, told of how they sometimes met in the bathroom of their doctor's office so that the wife could help her husband to provide the physician with a fresh sample of sperm. This particular couple is blessed with a great sense of humor, and they sometimes get mad fits of laughter when engaged in such highly unconventional activity. But such high spirits are rare. Infertility problems are fraught with so many deep emotions and guilt feelings that the subject itself often becomes taboo as a topic of conversation. Few couples manage to preserve their good humor.

The treatment of infertility—even if the problem happens to be caused entirely by female factors—can often result in temporary impotence on the part of the husband. In her relatively short career Miriam Biddelman says she has heard more about the failure of normally potent men to have an erection than most psychiatrists encounter in a lifetime. Reassurance that such failures are normal is one of the functions of the group.

Some infertility patients say that they have had a premonition about their problem. One young woman—whom we shall call Barbara—had been having sexual relations with her future husband Steven for two years without using any form of contraception. After they had been married another three years, they decided it was about time they found out what was wrong.

Barbara's problem turned out to be adhesions around the Fallopian tubes and ovaries. The adhesions were finally removed in what fortunately turned out to be a rather simple operation. She was then told that her chances had improved from 10–20 percent to about 70 percent, so she and Steven are still trying, hoping, and waiting.

Barbara's feelings fluctuate. Sometimes she is very depressed. At other times she can't believe that, as she says, "such a thing is happening to me when all my friends seem to be as fertile as anything. None of them tried more than three or four months before it happened," she adds with a mixture of resignation and envy. Sometimes Barbara feels as if there is no justice in the world.

"I was fortunate enough to be able to join a counseling group and that helped tremendously. It really gives me a lot of support to sit around with other women who have the same problem. It is very, very important," she stressed, "because the whole experience is a very lonely business."

Most patients feel that once they start to do something about their problem, such as taking one of the new fertility pills or undergoing reparative surgery, they become very hopeful about their chances of achieving pregnancy. Some think that to do otherwise would be harming their chances for conception.

"The disappointment after psyching oneself up in such a way is tremendous," one woman reported. (A postoperative or postprocedural depression after an initial high is a common occurrence.)

"When my body tells me that I am about to menstruate I get very, very depressed," she said. "Once my husband and I were out to dinner," she remembered, "and there I was in the middle of this fancy restaurant, and I started to cry. I just could not stop."

Grief is not the only emotion plaguing infertility patients; another is doubt. "One just has so much time to think about whether or not to have children," another patient reported. "One starts to wonder whether a child is really worth all that. After all today there is a choice, and there are all these presumably fertile couples who weigh whether they should or should not have children. My husband and I have become very spoiled, and even though we are trying our best to have that baby, we sometimes wonder what a child would do to our relationship."

Another patient too felt that all the waiting is most oppressive. "You go to the doctor every month. Then you wait to midcycle, then you wait some more. When you go back to the doctor he really does not have much time to talk to you, and since he is very busy he does not understand this time element. Besides all the procedures you undergo make you feel like a guinea pig."

Women in the "infertility group" have different opinions as to what pregnancy will mean. Some feel very strongly that they want to experience the growth of a child in their womb; to others pregnancy is secondary to parenthood itself. But all the members are frustrated by not being able to "perform" fully as women.

Sometimes, though rarely, the group helps a patient realize that perhaps she really did not want children after all. There are a number of patients who go through the painstaking infertility workup but at the end minimize their chances of conception by forgetting to take their medication, or to measure their temperature at the most crucial time of the month. If such "forgetfulness" happens too often it may be related to the fact that these women are often trying to become pregnant to conform to society or to please their husbands, parents, or parents-in-law. The group helps such patients realize that today parenthood is becoming a matter of free choice.

Most infertility patients discover their problem gradually over a period of months and years. For some it becomes a sudden reality—after emergency surgery, for instance. Sometimes this sudden knowledge is easier to bear because the operation itself was preceded by tremendous anxiety about the ultimate health of one of the partners.

One young woman, who had rapidly grown fibroid tumors that resulted in a hysterectomy almost on an emergency basis, reported that both she and her husband believed she had cancer. The relief Paula and Michael felt when the tumors proved to be benign far outweighed the eventual shock of knowing that they never would be able to have children.

Another young woman, who lost both ovaries because of acute pelvic inflammatory disease, reacted to her loss with acute grief. "I had always looked forward to motherhood, and then when I woke up from the anesthesia I knew that this would never be. I was swept away with loss, and many of the people who came to see me in the hospital made it worse. Some suggested that I was not the mothering type anyway; others came to tell me how hateful their children were; others suggested that I could always adopt. Most of my visitors, including the physicians, were singularly depressing and unhelpful."

For patients who are in the throes of coping with the possibility of being infertile, it may be hard to believe that some months or some years hence they will look upon their struggle with pain but detachment.

Very few persons ever lead a totally charmed life, and most of us are able to cope eventually with obstacles that at first seemed insurmountable. Couples who forever remain defeated by their childlessness might perhaps have been broken by another inevitable life situation. This does not make the situation any easier, but it is good to know that most couples will be able to handle their problem from both an emotional and a practical point of view.

Many couples who came to realize that their union would remain barren report that their marriage in time became particularly strong and satisfying. Some report that they live for one another, others enjoy indulging themselves, many somehow manage to put children, or young people, into their lives.

In times past, when adoption was easy, many prospective parents felt that a quick adoption would enable them to get over the disappointment of not being able to have their own child. Unfortunately this is only partly true. Adoption resolves childlessness. The couple still must make peace with the fact that they cannot bear their own children.

Actually adoption can mask the fact that the feelings of inadequacy that often accompany infertility have not been resolved. Many adoption agencies will only place children with couples who have gotten over the hurt of being barren.

Better contraception methods and freely available abortions have reduced the number of available babies. Miriam Biddelman reported on how angry many of her patients are at the pill, although most realize that an unwanted child is as serious a problem as not being able to have one.

Most people know someone who has been adopted, or a couple who adopted a child; they realize that these families are not very different from the more common brand. Adopted children, like natural ones, bring their parents the familiar mixture of joy and grief.

Not every couple wants to, or can, adopt. Some people —it usually is only one of the partners—just do not feel right about adopting, though when asked for their reasons they cannot put their finger on why they feel that they would not be able to accept somebody else's child.

One man, whose wife lost her ovaries in her twenties, felt that in his then precarious financial situation he could not possibly assume responsibility for another human being. The fact that this couple would have been equally burdened financially had they been successful in achieving pregnancy never occurred to him then.

Many childless women work and have more successful careers than would have been possible if they had been able to achieve motherhood. But at the time a couple is attempting to conceive, a woman's career in no way compensates for the pain and emptiness of a childless marriage.

Later, when the wounds have healed, many couples are happy with the fact that the woman has found a secure niche in what until recently was a man's world. The dividends of this lifestyle, even if it was a matter of necessity rather than of choice, come when the couple are in their forties and see their friends go through the empty-nest syndrome. Some women nevertheless remain ambivalent about their professional achievements.

The earliest years of childlessness are the hardest, when the houses of family and friends are filled with children, toys, diapers, birthday parties, and overwork.

Some of the couples who weather their infertility problem successfully manage to establish a secure relationship with other people's children.

Christine, the young lady who had always looked forward to motherhood but lost both her ovaries, adopted a twelve-year-old boy for a number of months. This made her realize, as she put it, that "one can love children who are not of one's body." She is still resentful that today with the real problems of overpopulation and famine, people with an infertility problem are often denied a chance to work through their own personal loss. This grief does not only apply to married couples.

A year after her own operation Christine has made peace with her fate: "For me there is a strong spiritual belief that everything in life happens for a reason," she said. "I assume that my mothering energy was meant to be spent in different ways. The only time I still hurt is when one of my friends is pregnant," she added a little sadly.

Paula—the woman who had the hysterectomy—also came to terms with her problem. First and foremost she and her husband were relieved that she was well and that they could continue to make their life together.

"We had not decided whether or not we wanted children and figured that we had a few years until we had to decide. Then we had no option left. The day I came to realize that I was less in control of my life than I had been before, I had to sit down and figure things out for myself." Here are some of her thoughts:

"From the time I was very young I had always been able to communicate with children and I knew that I loved them very much. When I did all that deep thinking, I tried to remember what my goal in relation to children had been. I remembered that when I was a sophomore in high school I had this fantasy that someday I would run this big orphanage for all those children in the world that nobody wanted. In my youth I fantasized a lot about all that. When I tried to come to terms with my infertility problems, I realized that all my early plans had revolved around children who were born to somebody else.

"I made these reflections over a long period of time, asking myself what it all meant, and in time it fell into place.

"Michael and I deliberately decided to become more involved with our nieces and nephews and do things with them. It is almost like being grandparents. We get all the pleasure and do not have the heavy responsibility. We spend a lot of time with them. They come in different ages, from two up to eighteen, so we get involved with all the different developmental stages. It's fun.

"We also have close friends who have a little boy and a little girl. Again we are involved with both the parents and the children, and we are the kids' guardians.

"We decided against adopting, not because of any psychological feelings on our part, but because it has become practically impossible to do this legally. We have some friends who sort-of bought their children and now they are constantly afraid that the biological mother will show up and make trouble. We just don't want to go through that. Our need is not that great."

Barbara—the young woman who now hopes that tuboplasty will enable her to become a mother—is at the height of her attempt to overcome her infertility. Though she has been living with her problem for three years, she says that she knows that her "worst hour is still to come." This is her first postoperative month. Her hopes are very high. Yet she fears that her body will let her know she is about to menstruate. Even though her husband Steven, like many men, wants children very much, she feels that an infertility problem is always worse for the woman, "because men just do not go through the monthly waiting and hoping."

Couples often disagree on how to resolve their infertility. Should they adopt? Should they resort to artificial insemination? Should one of the partners undergo surgery? These discussions can frequently result in feelings of resentment and guilt.

Barbara reports that her marriage has really gained strength. "Now we have a terrific relationship," she said, "even though at one point this thing was tearing us apart. We have so much time together and some extra cash. And we spend both our time and our money very, very pleasantly.

"Yet I am still very anxious to overcome our infertility. It is a personal thing, a challenge, a goal. I want so much to do this for me and my husband, I want this child to be part of him and part of me.

"I have heard of one woman who went through twenty operations. We all have our limit as to how much we are willing to do. I had my operation. I will not go any further; I am going to do my very best for the next six months, then I will solve my problem otherwise. I might be able to adopt a child then. I am not yet ready at this point. Now I am still concentrating on having our child."

Even after her tuboplasty, Barbara still works nearly full time at attempting to become a mother. In a defiant tone she said: "I am still taking my temperature every morning. I have been taking it every morning for three years. Twice I broke my thermometer, probably because I was so mad. It is most frustrating to live like that. You can't get out of bed and go to the bathroom without shoving that thing in your mouth for three minutes.

"A lot of times you have to have sex when you don't want to—and it's not as terrific as it could be. Fortunately my husband is a doll about it all, but I still wish it was over.

"It is very important to be working with a doctor who is encouraging," she stressed, pointing out that she changed doctors when she realized that the one she was going to did not hold out much hope for her.

Barbara also feels that counseling is a very important part of the treatment of her infertility.

Because there are very few specialized social workers like Miriam Biddelman, Barbara advises patients to get together on their own and share their problems.

"It always helps to talk to a friend about your problem, but nothing can replace the comfort of getting together with somebody who is in the same boat, who understands what it means to hope every month, only to be betrayed again by nature."

There is great hope today in America for patients with infertility problems. Not only is the scientific community interested in solving the problems of both the overfertile and the infertile, but in all fields of medicine there is great emphasis on self-help groups for patients like those functioning at the New York Fertility Research Foundation and the Boston Hospital for Women. If your community does not have a readymade group, you may be able to form your own by contacting infertility specialists in your area, getting in touch with the local chapter of Planned Parenthood, or Resolve, Inc., P.O. Box 274, Belmont, Mass., 02178.

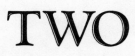

TWO

THE MAN

3

THE MALE
ORGANS OF
REPRODUCTION

And God created man in His own image,
in the image of God He created him;
male and female He created them.

—Genesis 1:27

THERE IS MUCH TALK ABOUT SEX ROLES TODAY, BUT THE MOST HEATED
battle along these lines was actually settled in 1861, when it
was finally understood that during conception one cell—an
ovum—provided by the woman merges with one cell—a spermatozoon—provided by the man.

Until shortly before that time scientists were divided into
two camps: the ovolists and the spermatists.

The ovolists held that since it was the mother who carried
the child through nine months of pregnancy, it was likely that
she also provided the ovum from which the child was to grow.

The spermatists held that the ejaculate of the man contained the blueprint from which the child was to develop. The
role of the woman, one illustrious scientist thought, was like the
soil in which the seed could grow to maturity.

Sperm cells were discovered almost exactly 300 years ago,
in 1677 by the Dutch lens maker and microscopist Anton van
Leeuwenhoek, and his student Ludwig Hamm. They observed
microscopic organisms swimming about in semen specimen
that behaved like the "little animalcules" that had been spotted

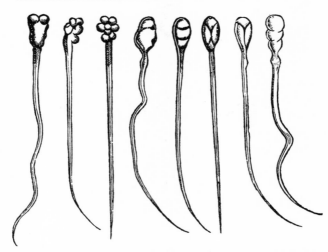

Sperm cells as drawn by Anton van Leeuwenhoek (New York Academy of Medicine)

in pondwater and various other biological fluids. The Dutch scientists correctly assumed that these "little creatures" had to enter the female tract before pregnancy could occur, and they named them spermatozoa or seed animals.

One reason why the theory of the spermatists was so attractive is that both the semen and the reproductive organs of the man are immediately apparent.

The male sex organs are mostly located outside the pelvic cavity. The physiological reason for their precarious, unprotected location is that the inside of the body is too warm for proper sperm formation.

The reproductive apparatus of the man consists of the penis, the testicles enclosed in the scrotal sac, several accessory glands, and an elaborate system of ducts, conduits, and valves.

At birth the upper portion of the penis is covered by a hood, also called prepuce or foreskin. This loose flap of skin is often removed shortly after birth by an operation called circumcision. Originally circumcision was a purely religious ritual; today it is often performed for health reasons because it is much easier to care for a circumcised penis.

The penis, the copulatory organ of the man, introduces sperm into the woman's vagina. It consists of three cylindrical masses of spongy tissue. One cylinder, called the corpus spongiosum or spongy body, is made of soft fibers. It encloses the urethra, which must remain open because it serves as a conduit for the sperm. The two other cylinders, collectively called the corpora cavernosa—which means resembling a cave—are traversed by major blood vessels that fill with blood and make the penis hard and erect before and during copulation. A series of important valves regulate blood flow in and out of the penis, and also see to it that urination and ejaculation are separate, well-defined functions.

Erection and ejaculation are entirely under involuntary neurological control, though the process can be influenced by psychological factors.

The average size of a resting, flaccid penis is 3 or 4 inches. When excited, it lengthens to 6 or 6 1/2 inches and the diameter changes from about 1 1/4 to 1 1/2 inches. There are, however, many individual variations in size.

Also outside the body are the testicles, long known to be associated with fertility. Each testis is about 1 3/4 to 2 inches long and 1 inch in diameter, and is wrapped in several mem-

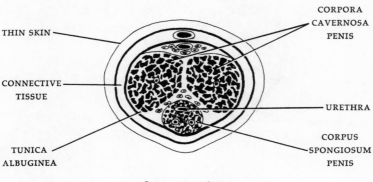

THIN SKIN

CONNECTIVE
TISSUE

TUNICA
ALBUGINEA

CORPORA
CAVERNOSA
PENIS

URETHRA

CORPUS
SPONGIOSUM
PENIS

Cross section of penis

branes or tunics. One of these, the tunica albuginea, is the toughest membrane of the human body.

The testicles are enclosed in the scrotal sac, a multilayered pouch laced with sweat glands and muscles. The sweat glands and the muscles act as a thermostat. In cold weather the muscles contract slightly to bring the testicles closer to the body; during warm weather the muscles relax, so that the testicles are further away from the warm body. The sweat glands also contribute to temperature control. The temperature inside the scrotal sac is about 2.2° cooler than that prevailing in the abdominal cavity. This is optimum for sperm production.

From puberty on, the testes produce enormous quantities of sperm cells. Spermatogenesis, as the process of sperm production is called, takes place in the approximately 800 coiled seed-producing (seminiferous) tubules that fill the interior of the testes. Each of the seminiferous tubules is about 2 feet long and as thick as a sewing thread.

Each spermatozoon starts forming at the outer edge of the tubule. During the forty-eight days it matures, it moves toward the center of the tubule.

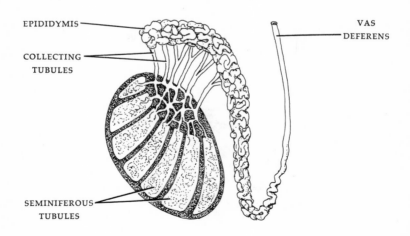

Testicles: From puberty on, the testicles produce enormous quantities of sperm.

Initially each sperm cell looks very much like any other cell of the body; but as it develops and passes through several stages, it progresses toward the hollow interior of the tubules and assumes its characteristic tadpole shape.

From the seminiferous tubule the sperm cell migrates to the epididymis, an 18-foot-long coiled tube that lies on top of the testicles. The word "epididymis" means literally "that which lies upon the twins"—the latter obviously being the testicles. The sperm cells spend several days in the epididymis, slowly progressing from one end to the other.

From the epididymis the sperm migrate to the vas deferens, which, as you can see from the drawing, is partially located inside the pelvic cavity. In function and in shape the vasa deferentia—there are two of them, one for each testicle—are very much like the Fallopian tubes or oviducts of the woman.

At its upper end the vas deferens widens and connects with the seminal vesicle in which the sperm are stored before ejaculation.

Although the testes continuously manufacture prodigious numbers of sperm, these only account for about 2 percent of the

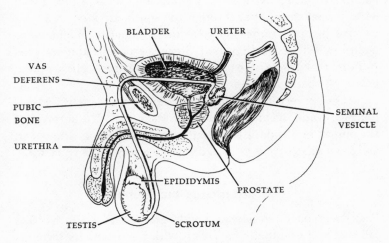

Major organs of male reproductive system

ejaculate. The bulk of the ejaculate is manufactured by the accessory glands, consisting of the prostate—a collection of thirty to fifty separate glands—the seminal vesicle, and the two Cowper's glands. These secretions together with the sperm cells constitute the semen. In addition to bulk, the secretions provide the sperm with essential nutrients that protect and nourish it after it is deposited in the vagina. Semen is rather alkaline—a property which helps to neutralize any urine that might be left in the urethra and also to overcome the acidic environment of the vagina, which would be detrimental to the sperm cells. It also contains large amounts of the sugar, fructose, of vitamin C, cholesterol, and various salts. Some of these components act as "spark plugs," putting the sperm into motion.

During ejaculation the average man emits some 200 to 400 million spermatozoa. These are deposited in the vagina of the woman and start to ascend through the cervical canal, up the uterus to their final destination, the Fallopian tubes.

Anyone who observes sperm for the first time is amazed at their number and rapid motion in the seminal fluid. They are reminiscent of the multitudes in New York City's Grand Central Station at rush hour. In a normal ejaculate most of the sperm are of the same size; they wiggle their tails in such a way as to propel themselves through the spermatic fluid in a purposeful manner. Other cells are more sluggish and move in circles as if listless or confused. Since sperm cells are produced in a constant progressive manner, some immature cells are present in all sperm samples.

Only a very small number of the sperm that start on their journey inside the vagina will reach their goal. The survival of the human race and the present population explosion, however, are proof that nature provided a large enough safety factor.

Capacitation of the Sperm

Each sperm has an oval head, a middle piece, and a long, hairlike tail that will eventually provide it with the means for locomotion. Compared to the ovum, the spermatozoon is very small.

It is nevertheless a very complex little creature.

Its head, called the acrosome, now appears to be a highly organized world of its own. In addition to much else, it contains a series of digestive enzymes that dissolve some of the protective layers surrounding the ova during fertilization.

Even perfectly formed sperm leaving the testicles are not ready to impregnate the ovum. They must first become capacitated as it is called technically. It is currently believed that the "spark" that enables the sperm successfully to penetrate the ovum is dependent on special enzymes present in the female genital tract.

Hormones

For the scientists, unraveling the anatomical structures involved in reproduction was only half the battle. As important was understanding how the body regulates the physiological processes involved in "keeping house" as perfectly as it does.

This feat is accomplished to a large extent by hormones. These chemical substances are secreted by the endocrine glands

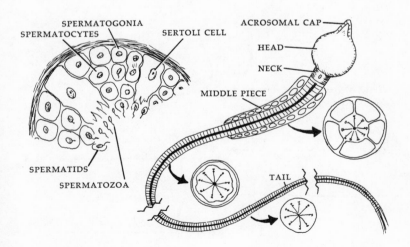

Even something as small as a single sperm can be highly complex.

into the bloodstream, which then delivers them to various target organs.

The best-known hormone probably still is insulin, which regulates the way the body utilizes sugar. People who lack insulin, either totally or partially, have diabetes—a condition that was usually fatal before insulin replacement therapy became available in the 1920s.

To be effective in controlling the body processes, endocrine glands often work in pairs by what is called "feedback." This mechanism, which plays a key role in reproduction and is taken advantage of in the treatment of infertility, works as follows:

Gland A makes hormone A, which stimulates target organ B to make hormone B.

Hormone B does its job (i.e., maturation of sperm cells, or ova). It also tells gland A that, as it is now around, gland A does not presently need to coax gland B to make more hormone. Gland A temporarily stops making hormone A. This step is known as *hormone inhibition* of gland A, or *negative feedback.*

When the level of hormone B decreases, gland A "wakes

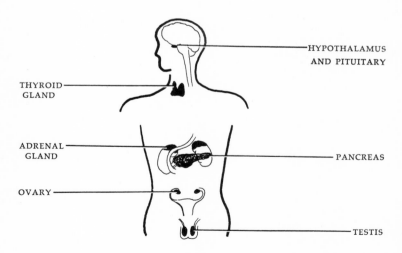

The endocrine glands secrete hormones that govern reproduction.

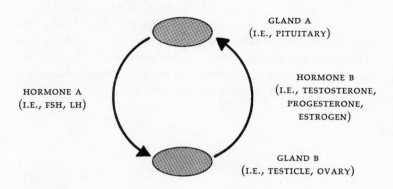

GLAND A
(I.E., PITUITARY)

HORMONE A
(I.E., FSH, LH)

HORMONE B
(I.E., TESTOSTERONE,
PROGESTERONE,
ESTROGEN)

GLAND B
(I.E., TESTICLE, OVARY)

Most glands in the body work by feedback mechanism.

up" and starts again to manufacture hormone A.

In reproduction, the major feedback pathway is between the pituitary gland (itself connected to the hypothalamus) which, among others, manufactures the follicle-stimulating hormone (FSH) and the luteinizing hormone (LH). Together these two hormones are called the gonadotropins ("tropin" means "directed toward"), because their targets are the sex glands or gonads. These hormones are identical for men and women.

At puberty the gonadotropins initiate the development of primary and secondary sex characteristics. In the woman they initiate the production of hormones (estrogen and progesterone) by the ovaries; in the man they initiate hormone production by the testes. Testosterone is the principal male sex hormone. In the testes it is manufactured by the interstitial cells, which are tightly packed among the seminiferous tubules. Testosterone is absolutely essential for the manufacture of mature sperm cells.

In the 1920s when scientists first isolated many of the hormones that control key body processes, they believed that they would be able to cure many of mankind's ills. Unfortunately the process did not turn out to be that simple. With its numerous intricate feedback mechanisms, nature is more superior at maintaining perfect balance than man can ever dream of being. But scientists are becoming skilled at manipulating some of these pathways. That is why throughout this book we shall constantly talk about hormones, hormone balance, endocrine function, and means of correcting hormonal mechanisms that for a great variety of reasons do not function properly.

4

DIAGNOSIS OF MALE INFERTILITY

The doctor may learn more about the illness from the way the patient tells the story than from the story itself.

—*Memoirs of Eighty Years*, James B. Herrick

Sperm Count

THE FIRST STEP IN DETERMINING WHY A COUPLE CANNOT HAVE A BABY involves a semen analysis. This test is important because men have been implicated in 30 to 40 percent of all cases of infertility. The test is also very simple, and thus if it is done first it can save much time by determining quickly the husband's role in the couple's fertility problem.

For a sperm count the man may produce a semen specimen by masturbation. Most doctors will provide the patient with a special 3-ounce glass jar into which he is to ejaculate.

When Anton van Leeuwenhoek wrote to the Royal Society in London about his discovery of the "male animalcules," he assured them that the sample he used was obtained during normal conjugal cohabitation. He also said that if his friends in London were shocked at his discovery, they should not publish this particular letter. Masturbation is still considered taboo by many and this can pose a problem when a sperm count is required.

Masculinity has for so long been associated with sexual performance and potency that some husbands at first refuse to participate in an infertility evaluation. Every gynecologist is familiar with wives who consult him or her about an infertility problem and state that their husbands won't furnish a semen specimen for analysis. Eventually most husbands will cooperate, though very occasionally a postcoital test (see Chapter 8) will have to be used instead of a regular sperm count.

Today most patients who have their fertility tested do not object to supplying a sample by masturbation. Male infertility specialist Dr. Richard Amelar has helped patients obtain a sperm sample by means of a specially modified vibrator. If absolutely necessary, a sample can also be obtained by coitus interruptus, but the results are less accurate because the initial portion of the sample, which often contains a disproportionately large fraction of the total sperm, may be lost. Sperm can also be collected in a special condom. But this again is less desirable than ejaculating directly into a clean glass container.

The full, tightly closed container should be delivered to the laboratory in a matter of two to three hours. It is important that information about when the previous ejaculation or intercourse took place and whether a portion of the sample was lost during collection should accompany the sample.

Some physicians recommend that the couple refrain from intercourse for five days before the sperm test. Other physicians feel that the time of continence should correspond to the patients' normal sexual activity. A period of abstinence of two to three days is usually recommended before a crucial sperm test. Long periods of abstinence reduce sperm motility and their ability to fertilize an ovum.

Since separate sperm samples from the same man will vary considerably in the number of sperm cells, a fertility diagnosis should be based on the analysis of two specimens delivered within a period of one to two weeks.

Spermatozoa are very sensitive to heat. Doctors recommend that if taken at home, the specimen should be kept before and during delivery at about 64°F (18°C), or the temperature of a cool spring day. The specimen should not be put in a pocket near the body, or near a car radiator (if it is delivered by car).

Once the sperm specimen has arrived safely in the laboratory, the volume of the ejaculate is measured. Sperm counts are given per unit volume, which is in milliliters (ml) or cubic centimeters (cc).

The sperm cells are counted in a hemocytometer, also used for blood counts. A small, measured amount of semen, diluted with fluid that will immobilize the wiggly little cells, is spread on the hemocytometer—a glass plate divided by grids into squares to make counting easier. Then the lab technician computes the total sperm content of the sample; the number of abnormal sperm cells; and the actual number of sperm present in each ejaculate.

The total sperm content of the ejaculate is important, but other factors count. One of the most crucial is the rate and direction at which sperm move (known as motility). Healthy sperm move forward head first.

In a test tube good motility lasts for only two to three hours. This is much shorter than the lifespan of sperm in the more friendly environment provided in the female genital tract. In the vagina, motility lasts for about forty-eight hours or longer, and the sperm cells themselves seem to remain alive for up to ninety hours.

Sperm cells must also be normally constructed—the scientific term for this appearance being *morphology*. There are at least six major types of sperm cells. There are the normal oval-shaped forms that represent about 85 percent of the sample. Then there are sperm with large heads, small heads, tapering forms, duplicate heads, tail defects, and abnormal midpieces. Since a man's ejaculate contains millions of sperm, it always contains some abnormal forms (about 15 percent). An infertile man may have a larger than usual number of abnormal sperm. Here is a table of sperm count values that are considered to be within normal range:

TABLE II
Normal Sperm Count Ranges

Volume: 2–6 cc.
Sperm count/cc. 20–200
million
Motility: 60–85 percent
active, one hour after
ejaculation
Morphology: 60–85 percent
normally shaped forms

And here are most of the terms a physician may use to describe the man's condition:

Aspermia: No semen. Aspermic men may be impotent; all are sterile.

Hypospermia: Ejaculate measures less than 2 cc.

Hyperspermia: Ejaculate measures more than 6 ml.

Azospermia: No spermatozoa in semen

Oligospermia: Less than 20 million spermatozoa per ml.

Polyspermia: Unusually large number of sperm cells

Astenozoospermia: Decreased motility of spermatozoa

Teratozoospermia: More than 40 percent abnormal sperm

Forward progression of sperm cells is measured on a still motile portion of the semen.

WHAT CAN BE LEARNED FROM A SPERM COUNT

A sperm count determines whether a man is fertile and whether the sperm are within the normal range so far as their shape, number and motility is concerned. Semen with 20 million or more active, normal sperm per cc. is considered adequate (see table).

Fructose

An important component of the semen is the sugar, fructose, manufactured by the seminal vesicle. The role of fructose in sperm capacitation has not yet been clarified, but its total absence—as determined by a very simple test on the semen—indicates a rare birth defect: the absence of the vas deferens and seminal vesicles. In such a case the testicles may manufacture perfectly normal sperm cells. These, however, have no way of reaching the outside world.

Absence of the vas deferens and seminal vesicles has the same effect as a vasectomy. It enables a man to have a normal sex life, but his ejaculate remains totally azospermic, consisting chiefly of prostatic fluid. The condition can be diagnosed very easily by means of a simple laboratory test.

Freshly ejaculated sperm instantly forms into a tapioca-like gel. In the absence of fructose, this coagulation will not take place. Lack of coagulation thus is an indication that the vas deferens and the seminal vesicles are absent.

Sperm Liquefaction

In the normal course of events the jelled semen will liquefy within five to twenty minutes. Failure to liquefy is another indication of trouble, since it prevents the forward progression of individual spermatozoa up the female tract.

All the causes for this particular abnormality are not known, but it is sometimes due to the presence of various antibodies (immune factors) whose role in infertility is just now becoming clarified (see Chapter 17).

Physical Examination

If your sperm count is poor, the next step will be a thorough physical examination. The physician will begin by taking a complete history, including questions about your past and present sex life. Do answer as completely and as honestly as you can. Anyone in the habit of listening regularly to personal problems very rapidly learns that no one leads a sex life as charmed as is depicted in the movies or the glossy magazines.

You will be asked about your job. Are you exposed to X-rays or radiation? Are you working in unusually warm surroundings (baker, boilermaker, truckdriver)?

Do you take very hot baths for pleasure or religious reasons (mikvah), or have you succumbed to the recent fad for saunas? Are you wearing tight underwear? (All these questions relate to the fact that sperm cells are very sensitive to heat.)

Have you ever had a venereal disease? What other infectious diseases did you have? Tuberculosis? Did you have mumps after puberty and did it "spread" to the testes? What drugs are you taking? (Some of these may depress your sperm count.)

Did anybody ever tell you that your testicles were not descended at birth or failed to descend during infancy? What about your weight? Are you a diet faddist or a vitamin freak?

Are you unusually disturbed about anything in your life besides your infertility problem?

The physician will also want to know whether you have a history of urinary tract disease, a hernia operation, or whether you underwent genito-urinary instrumentation which might have caused some internal damage to the vas deferens or the blood supply of the testicles.

Then there will be questions about your sex life: How often do you have intercourse? Do you find your wife unresponsive, and does this turn you off?

Problems associated with impotence will be discussed later, but certain religious practices, such as the fact that orthodox Jews must abstain from intercourse for a full week after complete cessation of the menstrual flow, have been shown to play a role in infertility. Some authorities believe that this law was meant to ensure that a couple would resume their sex life when the woman is most fertile. It works that way in most cases; but when the woman ovulates early, or has an unusually long period, the couple may miss the fertile days altogether.

After some more questions the physician will proceed to do a physical examination. Emphasis, of course, will be placed on a thorough inspection of the genital apparatus (penis, testicles, prostate, scrotum), but something can be learned from an unusual distribution of body hair and body fat, exceptionally long arms and legs as compared to the rest of the body build, and the size of the breasts and thyroid.

Depending on your general history, the results of the physical examination, and of your sperm count, additional tests may be required, including a testicular biopsy and a thyroid and other endocrine-function test.

Except for those related to sexual performance, most infertility problems in the male are reflected in the sperm count.

Persistent azospermia or oligospermia is usually caused by one of three factors: a disturbed endocrine system; impaired spermatogenesis; or obstruction of one of the ducts through which the sperm must travel before it can be deposited into the female tract.

Endocrine function can readily be evaluated by special blood tests. A testicular biopsy (see Chapter 5) is often required to distinguish between impaired spermatogenesis and obstructive infertility. Often both conditions are present simultaneously.

Sperm production may also be temporarily depressed by drugs, excessive external heat, or an illness accompanied by a high fever. In these cases the sperm count may return to normal of its own accord once the cause has been eliminated.

(Infertility may also result from a combination of male and female factors. These will be discussed in Part IV.)

Until very recently male infertility was an almost completely neglected medical problem. This indifference is perhaps reflected in the fact that andrology (from the Greek *andros,* meaning man), the medical specialty corresponding to gynecology (from the Greek *gynê,* for woman), is practically nonexistent. Men with an infertility problem usually repair to a urologist, a few of whom have become highly skilled in infertility treatment.

But times are changing, and treatment for men, as well as for women, is slowly becoming available.

5

CAUSES OF MALE INFERTILITY AND THEIR TREATMENT

For most diagnosis all that is needed is an ounce of knowledge, an ounce of intelligence, and a pound of thoroughness.

—Anonymous

Hormonal Defects

IN MEN, AS IN WOMEN, SOME INFERTILITY PROBLEMS ARE ASSOCIATED with a malfunction of the endocrine system. It is estimated that endocrine problems account for about 8.5 percent of all cases of male infertility.

Hormonal defects involve not only the sex hormones but also those produced by the adrenal glands, the thyroid, and even insulin.

Sometimes when the problem can be traced to a particular hormone, it can be remedied by providing the patient with additional amounts of hormone (replacement therapy) or by somehow decreasing the excess amount of hormone present.

Unfortunately matters are not always that simple because, as we have seen, hormones often work in pairs according to an intricate feedback mechanism. Low doses of clomiphene cause increased sperm production in normal men. Larger doses, such as those used for women, reduce the sperm count.

We saw in Chapter 3 that the pituitary hormones FSH and

LH initiate sexual development at puberty, and continue to be essential for the maintenance of adequate sexual function. Men who suffer from certain disorders of the pituitary gland often are infertile. But the condition can frequently be corrected by replacement therapy.

In general, however, the treatment of sexual dysfunction and infertility with sex hormones is still in its infancy. When testosterone became available during the 1930s, infertility specialists hoped that its administration would increase sperm production in oligospermic men. This unfortunately was not the case. Extra testosterone just instructed the pituitary to curtail the production of FSH and LH (the feedback mechanism). In any case, the net effect of the testosterone treatment was an even lower sperm count. Like its counterparts in the woman— the hormones estrogen and progesterone—testosterone just acted as a birth control pill.

When doctors discovered this effect, they promptly stopped treatment. But again surprisingly, after testosterone had been discontinued, the sperm count often rose to above pretreatment levels. Nobody quite understands why such a rebound phenomenon should occur, but it does happen, and some doctors give it a chance in men with borderline sperm counts. Other infertility specialists feel that the treatment can depress the sperm count for periods too long to warrant taking a chance.

Recently physicians have treated oligospermic men with depressed levels of pituitary hormones with human chorionic gonadotropin—a hormone produced by women during pregnancy—and hormones extracted from pregnant mares' urine. Promising results are obtained in about 30 percent of the patients. In view of the rapid advances that are made in hormone therapy, new developments are hoped for in the years to come.

Cryptorchism

Men with undescended testicles are said to suffer from cryptorchism, a condition that should be corrected during early childhood either through the administration of chorionic gonadotropic hormones or surgery.

Boys whose testicles remain undescended beyond the age of five start to exhibit some degree of permanent testicular damage, and testicular descent delayed beyond the age of puberty usually results in sterility.

Fortunately often only one testicle remains undescended, and most men with such a condition can father healthy children.

Thyroid Gland

The function of the thyroid gland is also evaluated. The concentration of the thyroid hormone in blood can now be determined rather easily by a number of tests, and the way in which the gland functions is tested by measuring how it takes up a measured amount of radioactively labeled iodine.

The exact role the thyroid hormone plays in spermatogenesis has not been determined, but both excess thyroid hormone (hyperthyroidism) or lack thereof (hypothyroidism) affect the amount of gonadotropins put out by the pituitary.

Once thyroid malfunction has been established, therapy is instituted promptly. Three months at least should elapse before the results of the treatment can be expected to show up in an increased sperm count. This interval is roughly equivalent to the time it takes for a newly formed generation of sperm to appear in the ejaculate.

Surgical Treatment of Male Infertility

TESTICULAR BIOPSY

Before a physician decides to attempt to repair an infertility problem surgically, he must distinguish between impaired spermatogenesis and various obstructive lesions of the vas deferens or the epididymis. Sometimes both problems are present. Inflammation of the testicles (orchitis), which can be a complication of mumps and other infectious diseases, can scar the ducts through which the sperm cells are delivered and also damage the seminiferous tubules so that they no longer produce adequate quantities of sperm. The state of the testicular tissue is evaluated by means of a testicular biopsy. The term *biopsy* always refers to the removal of a small tissue sample and its examination under the microscope. The physician whose specialty it is to look at tissue samples is called a pathologist.

The procedure is usually done in an operating room, under local anesthesia, although some physicians prefer a general anesthesia. If the procedure is done under local anesthesia, you may feel momentary pain during the initial incision.

Once the incision is made, a small sample of tissue (biopsy) is removed from each testicle. This tissue is then stained and examined under the microscope. If the tissue is normal, the trouble clearly is of an obstructive nature. If not, spermatogenesis could be arrested at any one of the stages of sperm development. The testicles may show evidence of being improperly stimulated by the gonadotropins.

LESIONS

About 8 percent of male infertility is caused by obstruction or absence of the ducts through which the sperm cells must pass on their way from the testicles to the male urethra.

We have already encountered the rare congenital absence of the vas deferens and seminal vesicles, which at present cannot be remedied.

Several other less severe problems can be corrected surgically. In view of the extremely small diameter of the ducts involved in sperm delivery, surgery is often difficult. But steady progress is being made because surgeons are now making use of microsurgical techniques.

The epididymis is the most frequently blocked duct. The obstruction can be present from birth, or it can be the result of infections such as gonorrhea or tuberculosis. During surgery the obstruction can sometimes be bypassed by connecting that part of the epididymis which is open directly to the vas deferens.

Today the operation is successful in approximately 50 percent of the cases.

The delicate vas deferens can also become blocked as a consequence of the same infectious diseases as the epididymis. Attempts at repair are successful in about 25 percent of the cases. Today the operation, which is called a vasovasostomy, is most often requested by men who underwent sterilization and then changed their minds. (The procedure used is described in detail in Chapter 20.)

VARICOCELE

The most common, and most successful, operation performed to correct male infertility is the varicocelectomy.

Varicoceles are varicose veins that occur in the scrotal sac. Such curled-up veins have been described as "feeling like a bag of spaghetti," by infertility specialist Dr. Karl Eric Johansen of the New York Fertility Research Foundation. Most varicoceles are large enough to be readily detectable by palpating the scrotum during the initial physical examination. The diagnosis of small varicoceles is more difficult, and the physician may ask the patient to stand up and lie down repeatedly while he is being examined. Varicoceles seem to disappear when the patient stands, and the different feel of the scrotum standing and recumbent may give the physician enough of a clue. The size of the varicocele has little effect on the outcome of the operation.

For some ill-understood reason the varicoceles form preferentially in the left side. This seems related to the interconnection of the blood vessels that supply the testicles and those that supply the kidneys.

It is also not known why varicoceles affect spermatogenesis. The static blood flow in the varicocele veins may affect the thermoregulatory mechanism of the testicles. They may also result in poor oxygen and nutrient supply to the growing sperm cells. Finally, some scientists believe that toxic material, which affects spermatogenesis adversely, may collect in the enlarged vein. Whatever the ultimate reason, or combination of reasons, varicoceles have been implicated in 40 percent of male cases of infertility.

Surgical repair involves removal of the enlarged veins and rearrangement of the blood flow in the scrotum. The operation is done under general anesthesia and usually requires four to five days of hospitalization.

Sperm counts have improved in 75 percent of the men treated and a pregnancy rate of 45 percent has been recorded.

Men whose preoperative sperm count was under 20 million per cc. are now often simultaneously treated with corticosteroids (man-made hormones resembling those produced by the adrenal glands) and HCG (human gonadotropic hormone) twice a week for ten weeks. This method of treatment has had favorable results in patients whose pituitary gland produces adequate amounts of FSH.

HYDROCELES

Inflammation of the testicles (orchitis), varicocelectomy, or other surgery can result in an accumulation of fluid under the thick tunica that envelop the testicles. Some infertility specialists believe that these hydroceles should be removed surgically because they interfere with the temperature control of the testicles. Large hydrocele sacs may also exert undue pressure on the testicles and impair the sperm maturation process in the delicate tubules.

Operations for hydroceles, which involve removal of the accumulated fluid, rarely improve the sperm count because most of these fluid accumulations are the result of diseases that may already have affected spermatogenesis adversely. A hydrocelectomy should always be preceded by a testicular biopsy.

Ejaculatory Disturbances

In addition to impotence or other sexual problems that are discussed in Chapter 15, men can also suffer from purely physical ejaculatory disturbance. The most frequent of these is retrograde ejaculation, during which the semen flows up into the bladder instead of leaving through the urethra.

Retrograde ejaculation can be a complication of diabetes, a side effect of medication taken for some other disease, or a complication of urinary surgery.

This rerouting of the semen is caused by a malfunction of the important little valves that normally do such a superb job at regulating traffic through the urethra.

Patients who cannot be retrained can nevertheless father children by artificial insemination with semen retrieved from the bladder.

THREE

THE WOMAN

6

THE FEMALE
ORGANS OF
REPRODUCTION

*It is of no importance that the ova of women are not, like those
of fowls, enveloped in a hard shell, for the latter are incubated
outside the body in order to hatch the chickens, but the former
remain within the female body during the development, and are
protected as thoroughly from all injuries by the uterus as by a
shell.*

—Regnier de Graaf, Discoverer of the "graafian"
follicle in which the mammalian egg matures.

MOST OF THE SEX ORGANS OF THE WOMAN ARE WELL HIDDEN WITHIN
her pelvis. The only part that can easily be seen is the mons
veneris—or hill of Venus—the small triangle of skin and fat
that covers the pubic bone and after puberty sprouts short curly
hair.

In order for the sexual organs to be explored any further,
the woman must recline and open her legs. Then the vagina
becomes easily accessible. Its opening is protected by a series of
fleshy folds, the outer (labia majora) and inner (labia minora)
lips. The labia majora are partially covered by pubic hair and
provided with glands that produce sweat and oil. The labia
minora are laced with glands that produce oil and also with
nerve fibers that are stimulated during intercourse. The outer
genitalia of a woman are called the vulva.

The clitoris is embedded in a foreskin and is located inside
the upper end of the labia minora. This organ of erotic sensation
is shaped like a miniature penis and consists of erectile tissue

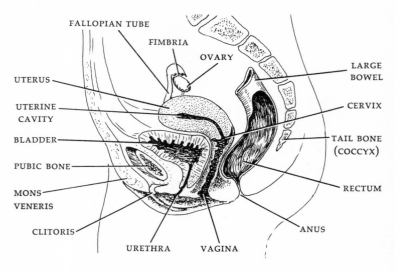

FALLOPIAN TUBE

FIMBRIA

OVARY

LARGE BOWEL

UTERUS

UTERINE CAVITY

CERVIX

BLADDER

TAIL BONE (COCCYX)

PUBIC BONE

MONS VENERIS

RECTUM

CLITORIS

ANUS

URETHRA   VAGINA

Side view of female organs of reproduction

and sensitive nerves. Appropriate stimulation causes it to become erect.

The clitoris of the woman, like the penis of the man, comes in all shapes and sizes, neither of which has a bearing on the pleasure it can provide.

The internal genitals consist mainly of the vagina, the uterine cervix (neck of the uterus), the uterus, the Fallopian tubes (or oviducts), and the ovaries.

The vagina is an elastic sheathlike canal that extends inward from the vulva and surrounds the cervix of the uterus. It is about 4 to 5 inches long and its diameter is variable. The inner surface of the vagina is lined with a delicate membrane that is sometimes covered with a film of moist mucus secretion.

In young girls the entrance to the vagina is closed off with a thin membrane—the hymen. The hymen usually ruptures quite easily upon intercourse. It may be so thin that it has broken long before that, but sometimes it is so tough that it must be cut out surgically. A small fleshy ring near the entrance of the vagina remains after the hymen ruptures.

The uterus (womb) is a firm, fibrous, muscular organ the size and shape of a pear. Its stem end is the cervix, which projects into the vagina. The cervix is about 1 1/2 inches long and can be felt as a firm round movable mass when a finger is introduced into the vagina. A small depression at the end of the cervix is the cervical os (*os* is the Latin word for mouth). This is the end of the cervical canal, the passageway through the cervix that extends into the uterus. The diameter of the cervical canal is about that of a thin soda straw.

The cervical canal contains many tiny glands that secrete mucus, which, as we shall see, plays an important role in conception—and infertility.

The uterus is suspended in the pelvis by several strong bands called ligaments. The uterus has strong muscles so structured that they can expand to accommodate one or more babies. The nonpregnant uterus has a small triangular cavity that normally can hold only a little more than a teaspoon of fluid.

The cavity of the uterus is covered with a special membrane, the endometrium—or lining of the uterus. Its proper development and healthy condition is crucial for the achievement of a successful pregnancy. The endometrium responds to hormones produced by the ovaries, and readies itself for pregnancy.

The Fallopian tubes or oviducts are the channels through which the sperm travel to meet the ovum. The ovum is fertilized in the end of the tube and is transported to the uterus for implantation. The tubes were discovered during the sixteenth century by the Italian anatomist Gabriele Fallopius.

There are two oviducts, one on each side of the uterus. Each tube is about 4 1/2 inches long. The tubes are funnel-shaped, and their open upper end has a fringed, trumpet-like appearance. Gabriele Fallopius called them uteri tuba (trumpets of the uterus) because they reminded him of the familiar musical instrument. But the name did not stick, and soon after their discoverer's death, the "trumpets" started to be called the Fallopian tubes. The fringes of the trumpet, the fimbria, are like

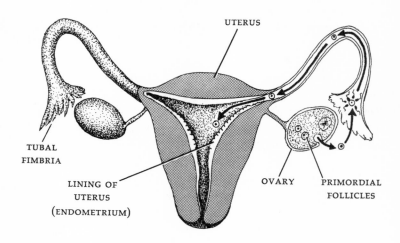

Schematic view of the uterus, ovaries, and Fallopian tubes

tiny fingers, and each is covered with a coat of microscopic hair called cilia. One fimbrium is longer than the others and is attached to the ovary to facilitate the transfer of an egg from the ovary to the tube. The tube is made up of muscles and fibers resembling those of the uterus. On the inside the tube is lined with a delicate membrane that secretes mucus. After ovulation the fimbria pick up the ovum and transfer it into the Fallopian tube. Vibrations of the cilia and contractions of the tubal muscles propel the ovum, which may or may not be fertilized, through the mucus-filled tube into the uterus.

The ovaries, like the testicles in the man, are the primary organs of sex, responsible for the primary and secondary sex characteristics of the woman. Each ovary is the size of a large olive. It is suspended in the pelvic cavity by a stringlike ligament attached to the uterus.

In the young child the surface of the ovary is smooth and pale. In an adult the surface becomes pitted with scars as a result of follicles bursting through the surface (ovulation). After menopause the surface becomes shrunken and grooved, resembling a peach seed.

The abdomen of a woman is a tightly packed cavity and the reproductive organs are not alone in it. The urinary bladder lies in front of the vagina and uterus. The rectum is located between the end of the spine and the vagina.

Hormones and Ovulation

Today every high-school student is taught about hormones, yet the first of these bio-regulators was actually discovered less than 100 years ago. The hormones involved in female reproduction were particularly difficult to untangle because the rhythmic pattern of a woman's menstrual cycle indicated that it must be regulated by a precise biological clock.

From this point of view women are not so different from other creatures. For many animals mating time is tied to the calendar. Deer and other forest animals mate in the fall so that the young are born when the leaves and young branches are at their most plentiful. In May of each year salmon travel across oceans, rivers, and waterfalls in order to spawn at the head of the same stream their parents did. In spring, too, birds return to their northern nesting grounds. Even though domestic animals have long since ceased to depend on nature for their food, spring is the time when barnyards, pastures, and stables are bursting with lambs, chicks, foals, and kittens.

Most animals have a clear set of signals that indicate when the female is fertile. A female moth, ready to mate, produces an odoriferous chemical signal (pheromone) that can be detected by a male moth miles away. Cows and female dogs too emit appropriate odors when they are fertile, which are recognized by the male of the species. Rabbits, whose reproductive capacity is legendary, only ovulate during copulation. The female rabbits must be able to interpret an internal body signal produced when the ova are ripe, since they only accept the male when they are ready to procreate.

A study of the human skin has turned up a few glands that produce a secretion that is unlike sweat. These "apocrine" glands, located in the armpits, around the nipples and navel, and in the genital and anal regions, are probably the vestigial remains of scent-producing organs that fulfilled a sexual function in our more primitive ancestors. Some day we may again learn to interpret and recognize these small signals associated with ovulation in women. Such a discovery would be a great boon to all those concerned with the problems associated with conception and contraception.

Once in a great while a woman is able to pinpoint the time of her ovulation through unusual means. Years ago a woman consulted the senior author with a severe infertility problem. She menstruated and ovulated only once or twice a year. She was anxious to become pregnant, but at the time there were no fertility pills or other means to stimulate her ovulation. After many a consultation the patient somehow recalled that before she menstruated she always developed a canker sore in her mouth. The little blister was interpreted as a signal of ovulation and intercourse was scheduled accordingly. The canker sore helped her achieve two successful pregnancies.

A few women also experience a stabbing pain in the pelvic area accompanied by cramping. This event goes by the German name of *Mittelschmerz* (pain in the middle), lasts for about four hours, and in rare cases can be accompanied by scant vaginal bleeding or spotting.

But most women are unaware of their ovulation. Infertility patients for whom the question becomes important must be taught to interpret the biological signs of their body.

These are the effects of the hormones that initiate and regulate ovulation and the menstrual cycle. The hormones play a crucial role in conception, and your understanding of how they work will be a great asset in overcoming your infertility problem (see chart, p 59).

Four hormones play a key role in reproduction; a fifth is produced as soon as conception has taken place.

The sexual maturation of young men and women begins when the bean-sized pituitary gland located at the base of the brain in the skull starts to excrete two hormones called the follicle stimulating hormone (FSH) and the luteinizing hormone

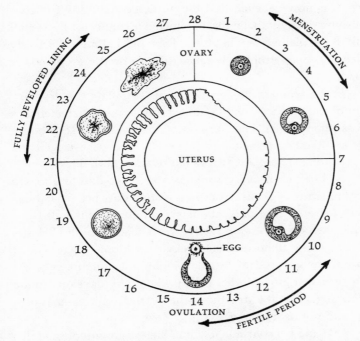

DAYS	GONADOTROPINS FSH	LH	ESTROGEN	PROGESTERONE	LINING OF UTERUS (ENDOMETRIUM)	FOLLICLE	CORPUS LUTEUM
1-5 MENSTRUATION	↗				SHEDDING	PRIMORDIAL FOLLICLE STARTS MATURING EGG	
6-13	↗	↗	↗		BUILDING UP	↓	
11-14 FERTILE PERIOD	MAX.	↗	↗				
14 OVULATION	↘	MAX.	MAXIMUM	↗		MATURE EGG RELEASED	CORPUS LUTEUM DEVELOPS IN EMPTY FOLLICLE
15-21	↘	↘		MAXIMUM	↓	EGG TRAVELS THROUGH TUBES	YOUNG CORPUS LUTEUM
22-25	↗	↘	↘	↘	READY FOR IMPLANTATION		MATURE CORPUS LUTEUM
25-28	↗		↘	↘	STARTS TO BREAK DOWN	DEGENERATED EGG	DEGENERATED CORPUS LUTEUM

Here are two drawings that indicate what happens at various points of the menstrual cycle. The arrows in the table show when the levels of the various hormones that play a key role in reproduction increase or decrease.

(LH). It is now believed that the pituitary gland itself is controlled by the hypothalamus, to which it is connected by a small stalk. As explained in Chapter 3, FSH and LH are collectively called the gonadotropins, because they act on the sex glands or gonads.

In the woman the gonadotropins stimulate the development of the primary (ovaries) and secondary sex characteristics (breast, body hair). The purpose of the ovaries is to produce eggs and the two principal female sex hormones, estrogen and progesterone. These are also called ovarian hormones.

At birth each ovary contains about 250,000 to 400,000 very immature egg cells or oocytes. Nature does believe in huge safety factors, since only about 500 of these cells will ripen during the woman's reproductive years. Each month FSH and LH, which like all hormones travel via the blood, trigger one or more of the oocytes to start developing into mature eggs. As each germ cell grows, other cells in the ovary develop around it, forming a cystlike structure—the ovarian follicle—that protects and nourishes the egg.

FSH and LH continue to stimulate the growth of the follicle. After about two weeks (day 12 to 14 of the menstrual cycle, which arbitrarily starts on Day 1, the first day of menstruation), it becomes "ripe" and appears on the surface of the ovary as a small bubble from which the ripe ovum will be expelled when "told" to by the LH. The oocytes that started to develop but lost the race to be first, dry up and become small white scars.

As the egg is growing, FSH and LH stimulate other cells in the ovary to manufacture increasing amounts of estrogen.

The pituitary gland and the ovaries, like many endocrine glands, work through a feedback mechanism. As the menstrual cycle progresses, the estrogen level increases. Noting this, the pituitary decides to slow down the production of FSH. Estrogen acts on the uterus and directs it to prepare a soft lining in case the developing ovum is fertilized. The endometrium responds and proliferates, and this portion of the menstrual cycle is termed the *proliferative phase.*

By Day 14 of the menstrual cycle, when ovulation is imminent, enough estrogen has been produced to cause glands in the uterus, cervix, and the Fallopian tubes to secrete large quantities of clear fluid mucus, through which the sperm can swim to meet the ovum.

From Day 6 on, the production of LH by the pituitary is on the increase. It is at a maximum ten to twenty-four hours prior to ovulation. Its job is to instruct the follicle to expel the ovum when it is ready, and to grow a special temporary hormone-production plant. After the egg has been expelled, special cells that remain within the follicle begin to grow and fill the cavity. These cells are yellow, and the entire cell mass is called the corpus luteum or yellow body. It produces progesterone, known as the hormone of pregnancy or gestation.

Progesterone makes the endometrium soft and delicate by stimulating the growth of many tiny blood vessels. Both progesterone and estrogen cause droplets of fluid to accumulate in the increasingly spongy endometrium, which will nourish the fertilized ovum. This is why this phase of the menstrual cycle is sometimes called the secretory phase. To make matters complicated it is also known as the luteal phase because it is governed by progesterone, which is secreted by the corpus luteum.

Progesterone and estrogen, which are absolutely essential for the survival of the fertilized ovum, also instruct the pituitary to stop making LH.

In the event of pregnancy, the estrogen and progesterone levels remain high, and gonadotropin production remains suppressed. If the egg is not fertilized, as happens most often, the corpus luteum loses its purpose. Its shrinks and withers, and progesterone production as well as estrogen production comes to a halt. Without their support the uterus sheds its now superfluous lining, and menstruation begins. Noting that there are no ovarian hormones around, the pituitary starts again to produce FSH and LH, and the cycle starts anew.

Over the years scientists have developed very accurate

methods of hormone analysis, and today the ovulatory pattern of women can be accurately deduced from the level of hormones in their blood.

A study of the chart on page 59 will tell you exactly what should happen when.

7

TESTS, TESTS, AND MORE TESTS

Diagnosis precedes treatment.

—Russell John Howard

DIAGNOSIS IS THE CORNERSTONE OF MEDICINE. DURING THE NEXT TWO chapters you will become acquainted with the diagnostic procedures used by infertility specialists. Not every patient will require every test. Details about the conditions uncovered during these studies, together with the appropriate treatment, will be discussed in later chapters.

As we have seen, few tests are necessary to evaluate the potential fertility of the male. But where the woman is concerned matters are not so simple. A routine minimal infertility evaluation usually takes five to six office visits. Most tests are performed in the physician's office; some of the more elaborate ones require a short hospitalization.

The fact that it is so much more difficult to pinpoint the cause of infertility in women than in men has its bright side. It enhances the opportunity for corrective action. Even with our present knowledge, infertility is much more treatable in women than in men.

It is also important to keep in mind that infertility often results from a combination of several factors, both male and female. A borderline sperm count, together with a minor defect in the reproductive system of the woman, may result in a childless marriage. There are numerous examples of infertile unions between partners each of whom had children with another mate—the most publicized being that of Emperor Napoleon I and Empress Josephine. Though their marriage did not provide Napoleon with the desired heir, each partner had children in a prior or subsequent marriage.

Infertility may also result from a combination of two or more minor female factors. Patience, perseverance, and a correction of all the factors amenable to treatment often results in pregnancy.

More than in most areas of medicine you, the patient, can become a full partner in overcoming your infertility problem. As a first step you must become very familiar with the complexities of the female reproductive cycle. Only then will you be able to follow the instructions of those attempting to help you. If you do not understand some of the words used by your physician, ask about them or consult the glossary at the end of this book.

The various phases of the menstrual cycle were explained in the preceding chapter. Review them from time to time; it takes a while to become aware of the small changes that play such an important role in conception.

In fact, the events that must take place from the time that the ovary sheds an ovum until the zygote (the fertilized ovum during its first twelve days of life) is safely implanted in the uterus are incredibly hazardous. Indeed, the favorable outcome of this perilous journey seems to many specialists such a piece of luck that the nine months of pregnancy that follow are by comparison relatively easy.

General Gynecological Examination

To start with, the physician will take a complete medical history and carry out a thorough gynecological examination.

Your careful description of irregular or painful periods,

the age at which you started to menstruate, any diseases you had during childhood, any spontaneous abortions, and the methods of birth control you have used may provide some clues as to the possible cause of infertility.

It is essential to secure precise records of all previous surgical operations. An appendectomy performed in childhood and long forgotten may result in adhesions about the pelvic organs that prevent conception. If necessary it may even be possible to obtain old hospital records, since these are kept for many years.

After the questioning is over, the standard examination will begin. Your blood pressure will be recorded. The heart and lungs will be tested for any obvious abnormalities. The breasts will be examined for lumps or discharge from the nipples. The region of the neck will be palpated so as to ascertain that the thyroid is not enlarged.

Then you will be asked to lie down on the familiar gynecological examining table in what is called the lithotomy position—thighs widely apart and slightly elevated in stirrups. Try to relax.

Your physician spends most of his or her working day looking at the insides of women. Relaxation not only makes the procedure more pleasant for you, but it softens your strong abdominal muscles and permits the physician to examine you more thoroughly.

The walls of the vagina are then gently dilated with a speculum, consisting of two smooth, curved interlocking metal or plastic blades. Now the physician can examine the inside of the vagina and see the cervix and the opening of the cervical canal.

During the initial examination the physician will do a "Pap smear" by collecting a few cells from the upper vagina, the inside of the cervical os, and the cervix proper. When examined by a specialized laboratory technique, these few cells will give accurate information as to whether you may have early cervical cancer. The test is so simple and accurate that it is now done routinely on all women. A smear to detect various infectious microorganisms is also taken at this time.

This is as far as seeing is concerned. From now on the physician must palpate. For a proper examination the physician will need to use both hands. One or two fingers of one hand are introduced into the vagina, while the other hand is gently placed on the outside of the abdomen.

Palpating gives some information about the size of the uterus, and sometimes about the ovaries. The Fallopian tubes, unless swollen or diseased, are too thin to be felt directly. Gross abnormalities of the ovaries and tubes are frequently and easily felt and distinguished.

More information about the ovaries—which have a tendency to move about the pelvic cavity—and the uterus can be obtained by palpating these structures through both the vagina and the rectum. Although it may not seem pleasant, examination of the uterus through the rectum can be most useful.

The presence and distribution of facial and body hair and pimples of the patient will also be noted. Both facial acne and abnormal hair growth may provide an important clue for a rare cause of infertility.

So far, you have just undergone a standard gynecological examination. Minor defects will have to be explored with more accurate tests; but a pelvic examination may reveal major causes of concern such as an oddly shaped cervix, a uterus that failed to develop to normal adult size or is tipped in an odd direction, major tumors of various kinds, ovaries enlarged by cysts, and perhaps even grossly enlarged Fallopian tubes.

A general physical examination can be done almost any time of the month. Since the female reproductive system works like a precise timepiece, most other tests must be scheduled. It would be useless to test for ovulation during menstruation, which occurs exactly at the opposite end of the cycle. (Physicians refer to the portion of the cycle when ovulation is supposed to occur as "midcycle.")

Some of the tests described in this chapter can be done over a period of a week, between menstruation and ovulation;

others should be done as close to ovulation as possible.

Cervical Factors

The cervical canal is lined with about 100 small glands, called crypts, that secrete mucus. During ovulation this mucus is clear and abundant and may even hang out of the cervical os like a tongue.

On the average a woman produces about 20 to 60 mg. (about a drop) of mucus a day. This amount increases 10- to 20-fold during midcycle.

The main function of the cervical mucus is to regulate traffic through the cervical canal. It can do this because it is a most unusual substance, able to form open channels within itself at ovulation time. Mucus also contain salts, fats, and sugars—all of which are believed to supply the sperm with some of the nourishment it needs on its long journey. The cervical mucus acts too as a reservoir for sperm cells, and allows them to migrate upward over a period of forty-eight hours or more after each intercourse.

Like almost anything else connected with conception, mucus production and its consistency is governed by the various hormones produced by the pituitary and the ovaries. Mucus production increases with an increase in the estrogen level of the body, and decreases with progesterone production. Just prior to ovulation, when estrogen production is at its zenith, the thickness of the mucus decreases so that it can easily be penetrated by sperm. In fact high-powered microscopy has shown that the long thin fibers of the mucus form definite canals at ovulation time, through which the sperm can swim rather easily.

After ovulation has taken place, when progesterone production is on the increase, the mucus thickens again. During pregnancy a highly viscous mucus seals off the cervical canal, acting as an effective barrier against sperm and various infectious agents.

It is easy to see that if the mucus does not respond to the

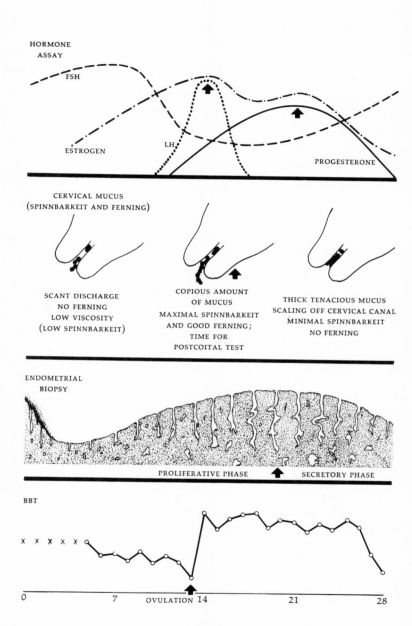

HORMONE
ASSAY

FSH

ESTROGEN

LH

PROGESTERONE

CERVICAL MUCUS
(SPINNBARKEIT AND FERNING)

SCANT DISCHARGE
NO FERNING
LOW VISCOSITY
(LOW SPINNBARKEIT)

COPIOUS AMOUNT
OF MUCUS
MAXIMAL SPINNBARKEIT
AND GOOD FERNING;
TIME FOR
POSTCOITAL TEST

THICK TENACIOUS MUCUS
SCALING OFF CERVICAL CANAL
MINIMAL SPINNBARKEIT
NO FERNING

ENDOMETRIAL
BIOPSY

PROLIFERATIVE PHASE   SECRETORY PHASE

BBT

x x x x x

0   7   OVULATION 14   21   28

Best times of the month (⬆) to investigate female fertility

6 8

commands issued by the hormones, one may have trouble conceiving. This can be established by two simple tests, both done at or near ovulation time, when the mucus should be thin.

One test is the fern test, so-called because normal, midcycle mucus dries in a pattern that resembles the leaves of the fern plant when looked at under the microscope. The viscosity, or thickness, of the mucus is another important feature. Normal midcycle mucus should stretch out twenty-fold like a thin elastic thread. This property of the mucus is called *spinnbarkeit,* which is simply the German word for "ability to be spun."

WHAT CAN BE LEARNED FROM THE CERVICAL MUCUS TEST

1—Whether the cervical mucus responds adequately to the ovarian hormones at midcycle.

2—Conversely, whether the pituitary and ovaries are putting out their hormones in a normal fashion.

Infectious Agents

The warm moist vagina is an ideal place for the growth of all kinds of microorganisms. It is estimated that about 90 percent of all women, at one time or another, suffer from some form of vaginal infection. Organisms called trichomonas and monilia are most common. Such infections usually manifest themselves by a copious white or yellow discharge and troublesome vaginal itching. These infections are not believed to interfere with conception in a major way. Their presence or absence is nevertheless ascertained during the initial pelvic examination.

In the event that one of these organisms is present, treatment with various antibiotics is instituted. Since such infections ping-pong back and forth between husband and wife, treatment for both partners is usually prescribed.

Postcoital Test

Practically all tests used to discover the cause of infertility are carried out either on the wife or on the husband. The one major exception is the Sims-Huhner postcoital test.

As its name indicates, this test is done *after* coitus (intercourse), fifteen to sixteen days before the next expected menstrual cycle.

Prior to the test—and to intercourse—you are to avoid douches or intravaginal medication for at least forty-eight hours. There is some disagreement as to the optimum interval between intercourse and the actual examination. Most doctors feel that four to twelve hours is near ideal. In any case, keep a record of the time when intercourse took place. When the woman arrives at the office, the physician will remove some of the mucus-sperm mixture from the upper portion of the vagina. The material is placed on a glass slide and examined with a microscope.

The postcoital test determines whether the sperm, penetrating the mucus, maintain their high rate of activity and motility. If the sperm are dead or extremely sluggish, and if the husband has previously been found to have a normal sperm count, it may be concluded that the woman's mucus is *hostile*.

Since the consistency of the mucus depends on the hormones produced by the ovaries, a poor postcoital test may be caused by a lack of ovulation. This fact would also be reflected in the fern test and *spinnbarkeit* of the mucus (see above). In this case the test should be repeated at a time when the woman is ovulating.

WHAT CAN BE LEARNED FROM THE POSTCOITAL TEST

1—Whether the mucus of the woman and the sperm of the man are compatible.

2—If the sperm are dead, or very sluggish, it may be further concluded that the mucus is hostile.

3—The cause for this hostility must now be elucidated. It may be due to lack of estrogen, infections of the cervix, or—in rare cases—to sperm antibodies (immunological factors).

Endometrial Biopsy

The preparation of the uterine lining (endometrium) by the ovarian hormones, progesterone and estrogen, must be in tune with the development of the ovum, and with the time at which the fertilized egg is expected to arrive in the uterus. If the endometrium is not perfectly prepared when the zygote arrives, implantation will not take place.

Again, the incompletely prepared uterus may be unable to sustain an implanted ovum for more than a few days. Such pregnancies may remain undetected; the patient might have a spontaneous abortion that also goes unrecognized and the ensuing menstrual period is simply characterized as being slightly delayed.

The healthy development of the uterine lining can be checked by taking an endometrial biopsy. The development of the endometrium for the purpose of receiving and nourishing a fertilized ovum progresses in such a precise, day-by-day fashion that in a normal cycle the pathologist can pinpoint the exact day when the biopsy was taken. The test, also referred to as "endometrial dating," identifies patients whose endometrial development is poorly coordinated with ovulation. This condition may cause pregnancy failure in women who are otherwise completely normal; today it can be remedied in most instances.

During the actual biopsy a few endometrial cells are removed with a straw-sized hollow tube that is introduced through the cervix. The test is one of the few used during the routine infertility investigation that may cause some discomfort. The patient may experience some bleeding and minor cramps after the procedure is over. An aspirin or other minor painkiller can be helpful, but most patients proceed with their normal activities.

The test is usually scheduled between the nineteenth and

twenty-third days of the cycle—Day 1 being the first day of menstruation—because these days correspond to the time the ovum is scheduled to arrive in the uterus. The biopsy can be taken at a later date in women with longer cycles.

Endometrial biopsies are usually sent to the pathology laboratory undated. The person who examines the tissue with a microscope estimates what day of the cycle it corresponds to, for example, Day 20 of the menstrual cycle. If this date corresponds to the one arrived at by the physician from an examination of the temperature chart, and from the date of the last menstruation, the patient's endometrial cycle is in perfect synchrony and the uterus is ready to receive the fertilized ovum. If not, something is amiss with the patient's hormone production pattern and/or ovulation.

There is some concern that an endometrial biopsy may interfere with an established pregnancy, and some physicians ask couples to abstain from coitus during the fertile days of the cycle selected for biopsy.

Actually if a biopsy is taken on Days 19 to 21, the fertilized ovum will not yet have been implanted. In fact some physicians have reported that endometrial biopsies removed at a later date in the cycle do not affect pregnancy, and that on the contrary the mild stimulation of the biopsy causes the endometrium to improve.

WHAT CAN BE LEARNED FROM THE ENDOMETRIAL BIOPSY TEST

1—Whether a patient ovulates.

2—Whether the two principal sex hormones, estrogen and progesterone, prepare the uterus for implantation.

3—Whether this preparation is in tune with ovulation.

4—Occasionally an endometrial biopsy may reveal endometritis (inflammation of the endometrium as a result of infection).

Ovulation can also be pinpointed by means of a vaginal smear. But this older, more cumbersome test is rarely used today.

Basal Body Temperature (BBT)

Most of the tests discussed in this book are performed in the office or hospital by the physician or his staff. One of the most important, however, is carried out by the patient. It involves nothing more complicated than taking one's temperature daily with a thermometer.

Though this is simple enough, the procedure does become a drag, especially because it underscores, first thing in the morning, that for you, becoming pregnant is not as straightforward as for most people.

During her fertile years, a woman's body is governed (as we have seen) by the hormones estrogen and progesterone. Estrogen is produced by the ovaries during the first portion of the cycle while the egg is developing. Estrogen decreases body temperature. The day after ovulation, progesterone production, by the corpus luteum, begins to increase gradually. Progesterone increases body temperature.

The effect of these two hormones on body temperature can be measured quite accurately. Body temperature is low during the first fourteen days of the cycle until the day after ovulation, then it increases abruptly.

The temperature of most women before ovulation lies between 97.4° and 97.8°F (36.3° and 36.6°C). After the egg has been expelled from the ovary (ovulation), there should be a sudden jump of about 0.8–1.5°F to 98.6–98.8°F (or 37.0–37.1°C). This temperature is maintained until menstruation, when it again drops abruptly.

Often, but not always, a distinct dip in temperature occurs a day before the sudden rise in temperature. The day of ovulation is the day of the last low temperature before the sudden rise.

The lowest temperature level recorded corresponds to the

day menstruation begins. In the case of pregnancy, progesterone production continues at a high level and the temperature remains elevated.

Even though these temperature changes are dramatic from a medical point of view, they are really quite small and delicate. This is why the temperature must be taken before you and your body have started to respond to the stresses and strains of everyday living. Your temperature is lowest after a night of normal, restful sleep. This temperature is called the Basal Body Temperature, or BBT for short.

The BBT should be taken with an accurate thermometer which you must learn to read. Several special thermometers are available with a temperature scale up to 99.5. Their markings are plain, and easily read, with less likelihood of mistakes. The temperature can be taken in the mouth (orally) or in the rectum. The rectal thermometer is less likely to give an incorrect reading. (Rectal temperature is always a little higher than oral temperature.)

In either case you should take your temperature each morning on awakening, the same way, before getting out of bed. Make sure that the thermometer has been shaken down from the previous day. If you take your temperature orally, place the thermometer under your tongue for three minutes. Do not eat, drink, or smoke before taking your temperature. The thermometer is also left in place for three minutes if you take your temperature rectally.

Read your temperature and record it on one of the charts provided at the end of this book. Your doctor may also provide you with a chart that he or she has developed for patients.

A blank chart, a normal sample chart, and one of a patient who conceived during this particular cycle, are shown on the following pages.

1. To begin with, study the charts and compare the given instructions to the sample charts. Note that the days of the cycle are printed horizontally across the top and that the temperatures are oriented vertically on the left-hand side. The numbers printed on the chart correspond to CYCLE DAYS. The numbers run

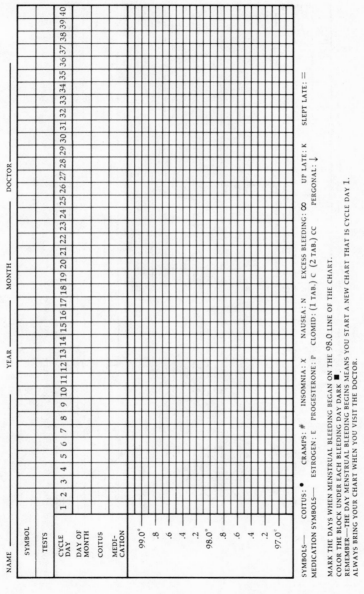

BBT CHART

NAME ———————— YEAR ———— MONTH ———— DOCTOR ————

SYMBOL																																							
TESTS																																							
CYCLE DAY	1	2	3	4	5	6	7	8	9	10	11	12	13	14	15	16	17	18	19	20	21	22	23	24	25	26	27	28	29	30	31	32	33	34	35	36	37	38	39	40
DAY OF MONTH																																								
COITUS																																								
MEDI-CATION																																								

99.0°
.8
.6
.4
.2
98.0°
.8
.6
.4
.2
97.0°

SYMBOLS——— COITUS: •   CRAMPS: #   INSOMNIA: X   NAUSEA: N   EXCESS BLEEDING: ∞   UP LATE: K   SLEPT LATE: =

MEDICATION SYMBOLS———   ESTROGEN: E   PROGESTERONE: P   CLOMID: (1 TAB.) C (2 TAB.) CC   PERGONAL: ↓

MARK THE DAYS WHEN MENSTRUAL BLEEDING BEGAN ON THE 98.0 LINE OF THE CHART.
COLOR THE BLOCK UNDER EACH BLEEDING DAY DARK ■.
REMEMBER—THE DAY MENSTRUAL BLEEDING BEGINS MEANS YOU START A NEW CHART THAT IS CYCLE DAY 1.
ALWAYS BRING YOUR CHART WHEN YOU VISIT THE DOCTOR.

a. This is a blank chart. Note the significance of the various symbols used.

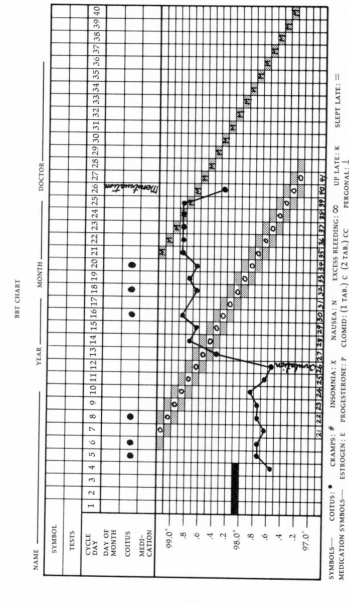

b. *Perfectly filled out chart*

BBT CHART

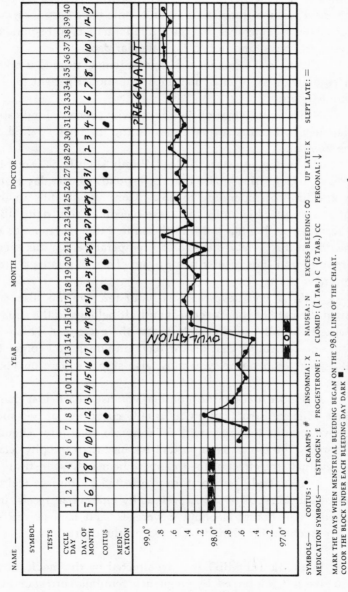

NAME ——————————— YEAR ——————— MONTH ——————— DOCTOR ———————

SYMBOL																																							
TESTS																																							
CYCLE DAY	1	2	3	4	5	6	7	8	9	10	11	12	13	14	15	16	17	18	19	20	21	22	23	24	25	26	27	28	29	30	31	32	33	34	35	36	37	38	39	40
DAY OF MONTH	5	6	7	8	9	10	11	12	13	14	15	16	17	18	19	20	21	22	23	24	25	26	27	28	29	30	31	1	2	3	4	5	6	7	8	9	10	11	12	13
COITUS								•			•	•	•	•			•		•	•			•	•		•		•			•						•			
MEDI-CATION																																								

SYMBOLS—— COITUS: •   CRAMPS: #   INSOMNIA: X   NAUSEA: N   EXCESS BLEEDING: ∞   UP LATE: K   SLEPT LATE: =

MEDICATION SYMBOLS—— ESTROGEN: E   PROGESTERONE: P   CLOMID: (1 TAB.) C   (2 TAB.) CC   PERGONAL: ↓

MARK THE DAYS WHEN MENSTRUAL BLEEDING BEGAN ON THE 98.0 LINE OF THE CHART.
COLOR THE BLOCK UNDER EACH BLEEDING DAY DARK ■.
REMEMBER—THE DAY MENSTRUAL BLEEDING BEGINS MEANS YOU START A NEW CHART THAT IS CYCLE DAY 1.
ALWAYS BRING YOUR CHART WHEN YOU VISIT THE DOCTOR.

c. Chart of a patient who became pregnant during this particular month from 1 to 40. (Twenty-eight days correspond to a normal cycle, but most women fluctuate a bit and some have very long cycles.) Always remember that the printed numbers correspond to your cycle days, and not to the calendar date.

Also note the dramatic change in temperature that takes place on the day after ovulation in the model patient in the sample chart.

A look at the chart of the couple who conceived indicates that they had coitus several times during the fertile period of the woman.

2. The day you start to bleed, if only slightly, is Day 1 of the cycle. Color the square that corresponds to that day black on the line corresponding to 98.0°. Continue shading in the squares on that line until you cease bleeding. Your daily BBT is recorded with a black dot in the square that corresponds to the day of the cycle and the correct temperature. Do this every day until you start menstruating again. Then you must switch to a new chart.

3. After you have recorded your temperature, also put down the date of the calendar month. It belongs in the square marked "Month" immediately below the cycle day. This will help you remember that on the days on which you forgot to take your temperature, you must also skip a square on your chart.

4. Be sure to fill in the month(s) you use a particular chart. Since your menstrual cycle will usually cover part of two successive months the entry will, for example, read July/August. Recording the month is important because then the physician can evaluate the effect of the treatment he may have instituted.

5. Your body temperature is affected by disease (colds, gastro-intestinal distress), as well as by emotional upsets, insomnia, late hours, alcoholic beverages, and lack of restful sleep. Such events should be noted on the chart.

In addition the BBT may be affected by the medications you take and, it is hoped, by pregnancy. Symbols corresponding to the more usual events—coitus, nausea, insomnia, excess bleeding—and to commonly prescribed medications (estrogens, progesterone, clomiphene, Perganol) are provided on the table.

Finally, bring your temperature chart each time you visit your physician. For the months or years it may take you to become pregnant, it is the "racing form" that helps you and your doctor to plan your future therapy.

The BBT chart may be used as a guide for intercourse. Remember that it only indicates ovulation *after* it has occurred. The BBT should be kept as a record of when the fertile period is most likely to occur.

Although the chart provides valuable information, do not let it rule your marital life. Since sperm live for about forty-eight hours, intercourse at least every other day during the fertile period is usually adequate. Intercourse can take place more often, if desired, unless otherwise instructed.

WHAT CAN BE LEARNED FROM THE BBT CHART

1—The BBT chart indicates whether the patient produces estrogen and progesterone at the "right time" of the cycle, and whether and when she ovulates.

2—The temperature chart reflects the effect of hormone treatment in patients whose infertility may be related to a defective hormone pattern.

3—After a patient has kept a record for a number of cycles, the temperature chart permits a rather accurate determination of a woman's fertile days. Fertilization is most likely to occur when intercourse is scheduled on the day before ovulation, on the day of ovulation, or the day after. (Sperm live and retain their ability to fertilize an egg for at least twenty-four hours. An egg lives for twenty-four hours. This results in a fertile period of forty-eight hours or two days.) Coitus should thus be timed to take place during the fertile period. It used to be believed that repeated intercourse decreased a man's fertility. This is not true. As a matter of fact regular coitus seems to have a favorable effect on sperm motility.

Since conception and contraception are like the two sides of the same coin, the temperature chart is the basis of the rhythm birth control method (abstention during a woman's fertile days).

4—A BBT chart is also important to gauge the optimum time for artificial insemination.

8

MORE TESTS: UTERUS, TUBES, AND OVARIES

Come, come, and sit you down, You shall not budge!
You go not till I set up a glass
Where you may see the inmost part of you.

—Shakespeare, *Hamlet*

FOR CENTURIES, EVEN MILLENNIA, THE INSIDE OF THE HUMAN BODY
remained an almost complete mystery because dissection was
strictly forbidden. In ancient Egypt, the belief that the gods
would punish those who dared defy this divine law was so
strong that the person whose job it was to remove the entrails
of a cadaver prior to embalming felt that he had to hide in the
hills after he performed his task.

The great Greek physicians had to guess at the shape of
various organs, or assume that the inside of man resembled that
of the animals they were allowed to dissect. Needless to say,
surgery was almost nonexistent.

Extensive surgery only came into its own after the discovery of anesthetics, which allowed the physician to operate at his
leisure. More recently the advent of X-rays, which help the
physician to see what needs to be done, and antibiotics, which
eliminate many fatal postoperative complications, have contributed to the continuing rise of surgery.

These diagnostic developments were of great importance
to infertility patients because defects connected with the anat-

omy of the female reproductive system also play a major role in infertility. Such problems must often be corrected surgically, but before surgery is resorted to it is crucial to evaluate the potential benefits that can be derived from an operation. The reason why the disorder occurred in the first place must also be established.

The normal shape and function of the female organs of reproduction were described in Chapter 2. The anatomical configuration of the vagina and the cervix usually play a minor role in infertility, but the uterus, and especially the Fallopian tubes, are a major cause of concern.

The pear-shaped uterus is a sturdy organ chiefly remarkable because of its enormous potential for expansion. Its shape sometimes causes infertility problems, the most common of which are "double" (bicornate) uteri, heart-shaped uteri. Various growths, including fibroids and polyps, can also cause infertility.

Whereas the uterus has a solid appearance and rarely develops problems, the Fallopian tubes can easily become obstructed. Such occlusions, as they are called, are one of the main causes of female infertility. Tubal malfunction results mostly from infectious disease, pelvic inflammation, and adhesions, which in turn are the consequence of infections, endometriosis, or abdominal surgery.

These diseases can also destroy the fimbria that participate in the transfer of the ovum from the ovary to the tubes proper.

One of the most important tasks in the diagnosis of female infertility is thus to determine whether the oviducts function properly (physicians call this a "determination of patency").

Four tests are commonly used to this end: tubal insufflation, or the Rubin Test; hydrotubation; a hysterosalpingogram; and culdoscopy or laparoscopy.

Information from these tests is considered to be complementary, though your physician may not find it necessary to carry out all four, unless some doubt exists after the initial tests have been done.

The Rubin Test provides information about the tubes only. The hysterosalpingogram supplies information about the uterus and the tubes; while culdoscopic or laparoscopic examination provides information about the tubes, the uterus, the ovaries, and, indeed, the entire peritoneal cavity.

Hydrotubation, during which liquid is forced through the tubes, also indicates whether or not the oviducts are open.

Rubin Tubal Insufflation Test

In medicine great discoveries are often based on very simple principles. So it was that in the 1920s Dr. I.C. Rubin, a great gynecologist who practiced at New York City's Mount Sinai Hospital, thought that it might be possible to determine whether the Fallopian tubes of a patient were open or closed by passing some gas through them.

This is like blowing air—or rolling a marble—through the hose of a vacuum cleaner if one suspects it to be clogged with dust. If the air, or the marble, comes out at the other end, one knows that the hose is open. If the air comes through hesitantly, something is not quite right; and if the air refuses to enter, the hose must be completely obstructed.

Dr. Rubin's test, usually done three to five days after the end of the menstrual period, is based on the same principle. A measured amount of carbon dioxide gas is insufflated into the uterine cavity. If the tubes are open, the gas will travel through the uterus and the tubes and escape into the pelvic cavity. If the tubes are blocked, the gas has nowhere to go, and only a small amount of carbon dioxide will be admitted into the small uterine cavity.

For the actual test the carbon dioxide gas is contained in a cylinder connected with a gauge that registers pressure and a valve that permits the physician to regulate the flow of gas. This pressure gauge is usually hooked up to a recorder, which traces the pressure changes on a piece of graph paper.

The physician introduces a special cannula—a small tube that looks like a soda straw—into the cervical canal, which is attached through a length of rubber tubing to the gas source. After it has been ascertained that there are no leaks, the flow of carbon dioxide is started.

At first the pressure increases; then, if the tubes are open, it drops sharply. If the tubes are blocked, the pressure will stay high. In the case of partially closed tubes the pressure will remain elevated, but it will not continue to rise.

After 80 to 100 ml. of carbon dioxide have entered the uterine cavity, the apparatus will be disconnected and you will be asked to sit up straight. If your tubes are open, you will feel a sharp pain in your shoulders. This is because the gas has collected under your diaphragm and presses on a nerve that is felt in the shoulders. The pain is sometimes felt in both shoulders, sometimes in only one, regardless of whether one or both tubes are open.

After you have felt the pain, you may lie down and relax until you feel comfortable.

WHAT CAN BE LEARNED FROM THE RUBIN TEST

If everything works perfectly and gas seems to escape into the abdominal cavity, it is safe to assume that at least one of the tubes is open.

A negative test, however, does not necessarily mean blocked tubes. False negative results occur. The cannula may have become blocked because its end was embedded in the side of the uterus, thus preventing the gas from entering the tubes. The very sensitive oviducts have a tendency to become spastic and constrict and thus block the passage of the gas.

Hydrotubation

Closely related to the Rubin Test, though used more frequently for therapeutic rather than diagnostic purposes, is a procedure call hydrotubation.

As its name implies, it means "putting water through

tubes." The "water" in this case is a saline solution of antibiotics and cortisone.

A small amount of this solution is put into an ordinary graduated glass syringe, equipped with a cannula that fits into the cervical canal. The physician pushes the plunger of the syringe.

If the tubes are open, the liquid will escape into the peritoneal cavity where it eventually will be absorbed.

If the tubes are blocked, either totally or partially, only a small amount of liquid will enter the uterus. The exact amount can be determined from measuring how much remains in the syringe or flows back into the vagina.

The degree of openness of the tubes can also be gauged by the ease with which the fluid flows through them. This can be determined by the amount of pressure that has to be exerted by the physician to push the fluid out of the syringe and the presence or absence of discomfort experienced by the patient. Hydrotubation is less painful than the Rubin Test because the results do not depend on whether or not shoulder pain occurs. Hydrotubation is used as a monthly treatment to help widen very narrow Fallopian tubes. The antibiotic and anti-inflammatory drugs dissolved in the hydrotubation liquid often improve minor tubal defects.

Last but not least, hydrotubation is used after tubal surgery to make sure that the newly repaired passage stays open.

Hysterosalpingogram

The Rubin Test is a useful procedure, but it only indicates whether the Fallopian tubes are open, partially blocked, or closed. It gives no information as to the nature of the blockage or its location. And it tells us nothing about the shape of the uterus.

The causes for conception failure are often multiple, and when the problem is refractory your physician will probably insist on having a more detailed view of your pelvis.

The obvious answer is an X-ray photograph that permanently records the features of uterus and tubes. But X-rays only record hard, solid structures like bones, and not soft organs such as the womb. This difficulty has been circumvented, not only in gynecology but for all areas of medicine, by the use of special fluid dyes that show up on X-rays. Such materials are called "radio-opaque."

A special dye is introduced into the cavities or structures before the X-ray is taken. Hollow parts of the anatomy, like the uterus and the oviducts, are sharply outlined.

Like the Rubin Test, a "hysterosalpingogram"—which takes its complicated name from three simple words: *Hystero* (Greek for uterus), *salpingo* (Greek for tube), and gram from *gramma* (something written)—is usually done three to five days after a menstrual period. Hysterosalpingograms are office procedures. The physician usually gives the patient a mild hypnotic drug like phenobarbital, and atrophine to prevent cramping. Both the bowel and the bladder should be emptied before the procedure is started.

When you are comfortably installed on the examining table, the physician (or the X-ray technician) will take a baseline X-ray. Thereafter 3 to 6 ml. of contrast medium is inserted into the uterus through the cervical canal by means of a special cannula attached to a syringe. The radio-opaque dye also flows into the tubes. Several X-ray pictures are taken. You may be asked to shift from side to side between exposures, so that the physician can obtain different views of your pelvis.

The first set of X-rays is developed while you remain on the table, or in the office. Depending on the results, it may be decided that you require more contrast medium before additional pictures are taken.

WHAT CAN BE LEARNED FROM THE HYSTEROSALPINGOGRAM

The X-rays will show the triangular uterine cavity and the Fallopian tubes which appear as two thin ribbon-like extensions.

Defects, if any, become apparent. The flow of the contrast medium comes to an abrupt halt if it encounters an obstruction in the tubes. An abnormally shaped uterus is clearly outlined on the X-ray film, as are polyps, fibroids, and other types of benign growths or tumors.

Unfortunately the hysterosalpingogram again does not provide a final answer. It gives us little information about the condition of the fimbria—the thin finger-like tentacles that play such an important role in the pickup of the ovum. It can also give no information as to the state of the oviducts on the far side of an obstruction. It says nothing about the nature of the obstruction; and finally it says very little about the ovaries themselves.

Culdoscopy and Laparoscopy

X-rays have their limitations. They cannot be used to obtain information about the organs located in the soft cavities of the body. Before making a major cut into the chest, the belly, the bladder, or even the heart, physicians have always wished they could peek first to determine what needed to be done, and whether there was any point to an operation.

The development of good optical instruments, including small telescopes, that could be introduced into a body cavity, was a major step in the right direction. What was still lacking was a light source so that one could look around in the "dark caves" of the body.

In 1805 Philip Bozzoni, of Frankfurt, Germany, projected the light of a candle by means of a mirror and a hollow tube inside the bladder of a man. Although he was successful and elated by how much he could see, his colleagues at the Medical Academy of Vienna reprimanded him for his curiosity.

The advent of electricity changed matters somewhat, and in 1878 Max Nitze developed the cystoscope with which one can inspect the inside of the urinary bladder. In this early instrument a light bulb was attached to the lens of the telescope.

The exploration of the peritoneal cavity came next. In

1901 another German scientist, Dr. G. Kelling, inserted a telescope into the abdomen of a dog through a small incision. The wall of the abdomen was then distended by injecting air. By moving his telescope back and forth, Kelling found that he could see the liver, the intestines, and the other organs located in the abdomen. The procedure was then adapted to human beings. It was called laparoscopy—*lapara* being the Greek for flank, or abdomen.

Laparoscopy has been used by American surgeons for several decades. During the procedure a small incision is made into the abdominal wall. A measured amount of carbon dioxide gas is introduced under pressure into the peritoneal cavity. By distending the abdominal wall and pushing back the bowels, this gas creates a clear space in which the physician can maneuver. Then a thin telescope, equipped with a light source, is introduced into this "pelvic space." The physician can now examine and even photograph all the pelvic and abdominal organs and structures.

In addition to diagnosis, the physician can carry out minor surgical procedures such as tubal sterilization and removal of minor adhesions.

Because the cut made into the abdomen is so small that it can be covered by a Band-Aid after it has been sewn up, laparotomy (minor or abdominal surgery) is often referred to as "Band-Aid" or belly-button surgery.

Even though laparoscopy was a major diagnostic development, many gynecologists felt that introducing the telescope through the abdominal wall was not the best way of looking at the pelvic organs. It was generally felt that it would be more desirable to introduce the telescope through the vagina.

From the beginning of this century some physicians managed to approach the pelvic organs through the vagina mostly for surgery, but occasionally for diagnostic purposes. It was, however, difficult for the physician to maneuver the necessary instruments.

As in the case of the Rubin insufflation test, major advances in medicine are often based on seemingly minor improvements. So it was in diagnostic gynecology. The vagina does not abruptly terminate when it reaches the cervix; its walls continue to rise for quite a distance beyond. The two spaces between the wall of the vagina, the cervix, and the pelvic cavity are called the anterior (front) and posterior (back) vaginal fornices. When the patient lies on her back, as she usually does during a routine gynecological examination, the vaginal fornices are almost totally collapsed.

But when the patient assumes the knee-chest position, as you can see from the drawing below, the posterior vaginal fornix stretches out into a smooth dome.

The senior author noted this fact in the late 1930s and started to explore the possibility of introducing a tiny lighted telescope by this route.

The procedure worked even better than expected because the posterior fornix has a tendency to balloon toward the peritoneal cavity when the patient assumes the knee-chest position. It becomes very thin. The intestines also shift out of the pelvis and a relatively large space is formed about the pelvic organs. This space permits the physician to view them directly.

Dr. Decker called his new diagnostic technique culdoscopy after the *cul*-de-sac of Douglas—the portion of the pelvis behind the uterus. The familiar ending *scope* (to see), as in cysto-

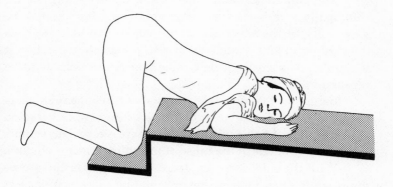

This is the knee–chest position. It is really very comfortable to hold.

scope and laparoscope, is used for many diagnostic instruments or techniques.

Originally the light source for the Decker culdoscope consisted of a tiny light bulb mounted on the telescope itself. Like all light sources it emitted some heat, which occasionally was troublesome.

A development in another scientific field—physics— eliminated this difficulty. It was discovered that when a light is shone into the end of a properly coated glass rod, it is transmitted totally to the other end of the rod from where it is dispensed. This property is preserved even when the glass rod becomes small enough to be called a fiber. In principle, a bundle of very thin glass fibers should be able to transmit a considerable amount of light, and since 1928 several scientists have worked at developing what today is known as "fiber optics." During the 1950s the method was sufficiently developed to be incorporated into the culdoscope.

Major developments making this possible were the coating of the fiber with a special material that prevents the loss of light from the sides of the fibers and a technique for spinning extremely thin fibers. These fibers are then carefully assembled into bundles that can be bent and twisted much like an electric cord. Fiber optic cords, carrying light into the remote recesses of the body, are now used for both culdoscopy and laparoscopy.

The importance of actually seeing the pelvic organs, including the ovaries and the tubes, cannot be overestimated. To a gynecologist the experience is not unlike that of a deep-sea diver who can look at the hull of a ship underwater and fix it if the defect is small, or determine that the vessel has to be repaired in dry dock.

Before making major decisions about treatment and surgery, the physician can now confirm good guesswork based on indirect diagnostic evidence. The procedure is especially important for cases in which the cause of infertility remains obscure.

With the culdoscope or laparoscope (together the procedures are referred to as endoscopy) the physician can inspect the surface of the ovaries. Are there fresh scars from recently departed ova, or are the ovaries encrusted with cysts?

And what about Fallopius's trumpets? Are the fimbria free-floating, as they should be, or are they stuck together and partially destroyed by disease?

Other tests have indicated whether the Fallopian tubes are open or closed, but now the physician can inspect the outside surface of these tubes. Are the tubes kinked? Are they flexible, so that they can contract freely, or is their movement impaired by adhesions?

The physician looks for evidence of old or active infectious disease, including tuberculosis and gonorrhea, that might have caused damage to the delicate Fallopian tubes. He or she will wonder whether that inflamed appendix was removed without complications—or were troublesome adhesions a result?

While the culdoscope or laparoscope is in place, the physician can improve inspection of the tubes by injecting some dye (indigo carmine) through the cervical canal. The dye will flow through open tubes immediately and escape into the abdominal cavity. If the tubes are completely blocked, the dye will accumulate on the uterus side of the obstruction. In case of partial blockage, the dye slowly flows through the tube after distending a portion of the oviduct before the obstruction.

Starch Test

Since the ovum must rely for transportation on the contractions of the Fallopian tubes, it is important to find out whether these indeed are able to perform their function.

The presence of an ovum can be mimicked by ordinary sterile starch particles deposited at the upper end of the Fallopian tube by means of the culdoscope. If all is well, the fimbria will pick up the starch grains and deliver them at the other end of the genital tract in a matter of twenty-four to seventy-two hours. Here they can be collected in the cervical mucus, stained with iodine, and identified on a microscope slide.

Minor Surgery

The culdoscope and laparoscope are mostly used for diagnosis. But while the physician examines the pelvic cavity, the instruments can be used to carry out minor surgery such as snipping off adhesions that kink the tubes or freeing up fimbria that have become stuck together.

Procedure for Culdoscopy and Laparoscopy

Most physicians prefer to hospitalize patients who are to undergo culdoscopic examinations. Other tests, such as a twenty-four-hour urine collection for hormone analysis, or a dilatation and curettage (D & C)—an operation during which the cervix is dilated and the uterus scraped out—are often carried out at the same time.

You will be admitted to the hospital the afternoon before the examination. After all the customary admission tests required by the hospital are over, you will have a regular evening meal. If you feel at all anxious about sleeping in strange surroundings, ask your physician whether you may have a sleeping pill.

Most hospitals wake their patients early, but once you are up breakfast is omitted for all those scheduled to undergo a surgical or extensive diagnostic procedure early in the day. This prevents nausea, which is not only unpleasant but can also be dangerous in anesthetized patients. Though it is not a fair exchange, instead of breakfast you will have an enema.

When you arrive in the operating room, the physician will explain how to assume the knee-chest position. Your cooperation is most important because this makes things easier for both you and your doctor.

The knee-chest position is comfortable (especially since the physician will use a table designed to make it easy). Many babies assume this position quite naturally for sleeping. It can be maintained without fatigue for thirty to forty-five minutes.

Relax. The procedure you are about to undergo involves no pain, cutting, stitching, or blood loss. It takes about fifteen minutes.

General anesthesia is unnecessary. Most patients are sedated with various combinations of Demerol, scopolamine, and/or barbiturates. Local anesthesia (Novocaine or a similar drug) injected into the vaginal vault is used to eliminate pain during the entire procedure.

During the procedure you will be quite relaxed. Some patients actually talk with their physicians, others sleep.

Air will enter your abdomen as soon as the physician punctures the cul-de-sac. When all is over, and the physician has lowered you on your abdomen, he will press it with both hands. This expels most of the air. If any remains, you may experience some distress in the shoulder region. This pain is relieved by lying flat, without a pillow. It sometimes helps to elevate the feet. Aspirin or another minor pain reliever will help if necessary.

The small puncture hole through which the physician has inserted the instrument does not require stitching. You can return home the same evening, or the morning after the operation is over. Douching is forbidden for one week after the examination, as is intercourse.

WHAT CAN BE LEARNED FROM ENDOSCOPY (CULDOSCOPY AND LAPAROSCOPY)

These examinations often provide a firm answer to many questions related to infertility, as well as to ordinary gynecological problems.

For our purpose the procedure permits physicians to pinpoint pelvic disease in women appearing "normal." It allows physicians:

1—To determine the condition of the tubes and ovaries; to confirm diagnosis such as endometriosis, ovarian disease, damage wrought by long-term infectious disease, and many other major causes of infertility.

2—To determine whether the oviducts are suitable for surgical reconstruction.

3—To evaluate the possible benefits derived from other types of surgery.

9

FERTILITY DRUGS

Everything depends, as in all human relations, upon dosage.

—Alexander Lenard

FEW MEDICAL DEVELOPMENTS HAVE BEEN AWAITED WITH GREATER eagerness than "the pill" that permits women to control their fecundity, and a fertility drug that permits the childless to bear children. To have or not to have has always been an important question for couples.

The search to cure infertility is very ancient. The Bible already speaks of the magic and aphrodisiacal power of the mandrake plant, which later became a chief staple of the medieval herb garden.

Celsus, the author of the one great Roman book on medicine, *De Re Medicina,* written about A.D. 30, stated that "lion's fat softened by rose oil would aid conception." And during the Middle Ages the abbess Hildegard of Bingen recommended that sterile women dine on the uteri of virgin cows and sheep. With some stretch of the imagination one might interpret this as a forerunner of hormone therapy.

In spite of the antiquity of the search, it is only in our own times that scientists have developed drugs to help both the overfertile and the sterile.

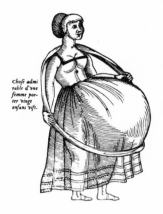

Chofe admirable d'vne femme porter vingt enfans vifs.

This woodcut, dating from 1575, is of a woman allegedly carrying twenty living children. (Courtesy of National Library of Medicine, Bethesda, Maryland)

To date all these agents are either hormones, hormone-like substances, or drugs that specifically interfere with hormone regulation. Even though these drugs are still far from perfect, they represent a major medical advance in solving problems that affect a large segment of the population.

Failure of Ovulation

About 20 to 25 percent of all cases of infertility are related to ovulatory failure. The reasons for this failure are manifold. In extreme cases the ovaries may be congenitally absent or non-functional, even though the patient may maintain all or most of her feminine characteristics. In less serious cases the ovaries are present but somehow do not manage to mature and/or expel ova, even though the pituitary gland seems to function adequately.

There are other reasons for ovulatory failure: overwork, chronic fatigue, disease, improper diet, and prolonged use of birth control pills. Pelvic infections following venereal disease are a serious and frequent cause for ovarian failure, as is peritonitis following appendicitis or other abdominal surgery. In these cases the capsules that enclose the ovaries may become thickened, and it may be impossible for the egg-bearing follicle to break out.

The ovaries may also fail to produce an egg because the two pituitary hormones FSH and LH do not work precisely enough to release an egg at the proper time. Too much or too little of either hormone produced out of step with the production of estrogen and progesterone causes such failure. Today ovulation can be induced in 80 percent of women who do not ovulate. Fertility drugs, however, are expensive and their administration is associated with a certain risk. This is why it is desirable to conduct a thorough infertility investigation before embarking on such drug treatment. It is also mandatory that the husband's fertility be established before they are used.

Clomiphene Citrate Therapy

We would like to remind you that the four principal hormones involved in female reproduction, the follicle stimulating hormone (FSH), lutienizing hormone (LH), estrogen, and progesterone work in seesaw fashion.

The gonadotropic hormones FSH and LH trigger the development and release of the mature ovum. This event is accompanied by a rise in the concentration of the ovarian hormones estrogen and progesterone. These in turn supress the production of FSH and LH. Production of the gonadotropins by the pituitary remains supressed as long as the level of either ovarian hormone remains high.

In biology such an arrangement is called a feedback mechanism. In the case of the ovarian hormones and the gonadotropins, scientists believe that feedback loop works as follows: The pituitary itself is under the control of the hypothalamus, to which it is connected by a thin stalk. The hypothalamus apparently has "special groves" (receptor sites) for each of the hormones whose concentration it controls, including estrogen. When the blood level of estrogen is high, the "estrogen groves" on the hypothalamus are filled with estrogen. This "tells" the pituitary to hold off the production of FSH and

LH. When blood levels of estrogen decrease, the "groves" on the hypothalamus become empty and the mechanism for gonadotrop production is set in motion. During pregnancy the permanently high levels of the ovarian hormones ensures an anovulatory state.

The feedback mechanisms that play such an important role in reproduction were not known some thirty years ago when gynecologist Dr. John Rock searched for a drug to help some of his infertile patients conceive.

He almost naturally turned to progesterone, the hormone of pregnancy. Progesterone did not induce ovulation; as a matter of fact it was shown to prevent ovulation. Man-made progestins are now widely used as oral contraceptives, and Dr. Rock became one of the three fathers of the birth control pill.

Science often follows a curious path. While Dr. Rock searched for a fertility pill and came up with a birth control pill, Dr. R. B. Greenblatt, also deeply involved in unraveling the intricacies of the human reproductive cycle, was looking for a contraceptive.

In 1960 he was studying the effects of the anti-estrogen MER-25, and to his great surprise found that it did not have a contraceptive effect. On the contrary, it stimulated ovulation in laboratory animals.

It often happens that the same discovery is made independently in different laboratories. At about the time that Dr. Greenblatt discovered by accident that MER-25 increased ovulation in laboratory animals and in human patients, Drs. Robert W. Kistner and O. W. Smith, of the Harvard University Medical School, noted that four women suffering from the Stein-Leventhal Syndrome (see Chapter 6), a condition usually associated with ovarian failure, became pregnant when treated with MER-25.

After several chemical modifications MER-25 became clomiphene citrate (Clomid), which has been used as one of the two currently available fertility drugs since the 1960s. So far nobody quite knows how clomiphene works. It is believed, however, that the mechanism is what scientists call "competitive inhibition." Clomiphene resembles estrogen so closely that it fits into the special groves of the hypothalamus which instructs the pituitary whether or not to produce FSH. Clomiphene occupies these sites, but—and here is why it works as a fertility pill—it does not transmit estrogen's message. So the pituitary goes right on manufacturing FSH. In fact it seems able to coax the pituitary into making more FSH than usual. This increased level of FSH often can convince reluctant ovaries to mature a follicle.

Clomiphene does not work for all women who fail to ovulate. First of all, the patient must have adequate levels of estrogen. Second, the pituitary must be able to produce FSH, and finally the ovaries must be healthy enough to produce mature ova.

The drug has been proved to work for patients suffering from polycystic ovarian disease. In such cases the extra amount of FSH might convince a ripening follicle to break through a somewhat thickened mantle. The drug is also suitable for women who fail to menstruate (amenorrhea) or menstruate infrequently or have scanty periods (oligomenorrhea). Clomiphene is also indicated for women who once were quite regular but whose menstrual and ovulatory pattern has become adversely affected through the use of birth control pills (post-pill amenorrhea). Some physicians also use clomiphene regularly in conjunction with artificial insemination to ensure that their patients continue to ovulate according to schedule.

Procedure

The routine fertility workup will have indicated whether you are a candidate for clomiphene therapy.

If it has not already been done, the physician may want to find out whether you produce adequate levels of estrogen. This can be determined by direct measurement of the level of estrogen in the bloodstream or urine; by means of endometrial biopsy; by examination of vaginal smears; or by giving you progesterone. The last method is based on the fact that menstrual bleeding follows the sequential production of estrogen and progesterone by the ovaries.

Women whose ovaries do not develop a competent corpus luteum often have inadequate levels of progesterone after ovulation. This in turn results in delayed menstrual periods.

Diagnosis of this particular condition involves the administration of progesterone either by mouth or by injection. Onset of menstruation within a week indicates that the ovaries at least produce adequate levels of estrogen. The condition often responds to clomiphene therapy.

Once it has been decided to give clomiphene a try, you will receive 50 mg. of the medication for five consecutive days, starting on Day 5 of the menstrual cycle.

Ovulation should occur five to nine days after the last dose. Your BBT chart will indicate whether in fact you did ovulate. If you failed to ovulate, the physician will probably increase the dosage level during your next cycle. This will be decided upon after you have been carefully examined in order to make sure that the clomiphene has not caused the development of unruptured follicles (ovarian cysts) or that by chance you may be pregnant. The examination is frequently done during your menstruation. Ovarian enlargement unfortunately occurs in 14 percent of the patients who are given clomiphene therapy, and preexisting ovarian cysts or a history thereof is a contraindication for clomiphene therapy. Most clomiphene-induced cysts regress by themselves.

Because it is an anti-estrogen agent, one of the minor complications of clomiphene therapy is that it may initiate the production of a scanty, thick cervical mucus. (Estrogen normally sees to it that the cervical mucus is copious and easily penetrated by sperm at ovulation time.) A scanty, thick mucus can make sperm penetration difficult. This factor can be checked out by means of a postcoital test, and the condition corrected by administration of small doses of estrogen.

To complete ovulation and expel the ovum from the ovary, some patients will need a small dose of human chorionic gonadotropic hormone (HCG), the special hormone detected during the pregnancy test, which we discussed at the beginning of this chapter. In this case the human chorionic gonadotropin does the job of the luteinizing hormone (LH), which it resembles so closely.

Unless there are serious side effects, clomiphene therapy is continued for eight to ten months. The drug seems to induce ovulation in 75 percent of suitable patients, but only 30 percent of those treated become pregnant. Fraternal twins (resulting from two ova) occur in 7 percent of clomiphene-induced pregnancies. There is no increase in the number of identical twins. The rate of spontaneous abortion is high (20–25 percent) but this figure seems to be unrelated to the length of clomiphene therapy. The drug does not increase the number of abnormal babies.

Excellent results are seen in patients suffering from Stein-Leventhal ovaries, and clomiphene therapy has reduced the need for surgical wedge resection that was previously used exclusively to treat this condition (see Chapter 10). The follicle stimulating hormone Pergonal is used in polycystic (Stein-Leventhal) ovaries only as a last resort. The risk of complication is greatest when the ovaries are large, with follicle cysts. But if clomiphene therapy fails, surgical wedge resection is recommended.

Therapy with Gonadotropins

Once it became understood that ovulation is initiated by the gonadotropins, it was logical to see whether a failure to ovulate could be corrected by the administration of the follicle stimulating hormone.

Two hurdles had to be overcome. The first was to find a source for FSH and LH. The second was to give just enough of the hormone. Hormones are released by the glands in microscopic amounts only. In the body there usually is another hormone ready to intervene as soon as the first hormone seems to have done its job.

To find a suitable source for FSH and LH, Dr. Carl A.

Gemzell, of Uppsala University in Sweden, started to collect pituitary glands from cadavers. The pituitary gland is very small and makes about half a dozen important hormones, so the problem of preparing enough FSH to treat patients was a major one. Indeed it took Dr. Gemzell a long time to purify enough FSH to demonstrate that the method worked. The FSH alone did not do the trick. At the right moment the patient had to be treated with HCG to trigger the release of the ovum from its follicle.

Dr. Gemzell reported his first series of successfully pregnant women in 1963. However it was already evident from these early results that both the number of spontaneous abortions and the number of multiple pregnancies was much higher than in normal women.

Indeed for a while it was customary to read of the birth of triplets, quadruplets, and quintuplets as if it happened every day. Yet the birth of quintuplets used to be so rare that the Dionne quintuplets of the 1930s made world history. When quintuplets were born in Holland in 1719 it also seems to have been a major event, and people came from afar to see the sight.

Extracting FSH and LH from human pituitary glands was difficult, and the hormone extracted from animal pituitaries did not work very well. Fortunately scientists began to exploit another source of gonadotropins. It had been noted as long ago as 1929 that the pituitary in menopausal women works overtime in an attempt to convince the failing ovaries to continue producing ripe follicles. The excess hormone was eliminated through the kidneys. The urine of these women thus contains much higher concentrations of FSH and LH than normal. Attempts at isolating these hormones were finally successful in 1961, and the product was marketed under the trade name of Pergonal. It must be used in conjunction with HCG.

The hormone FSH, extracted from the pituitary gland of cadavers, is referred to as HPG (Hormone Pituitary Gonadotropin).

Pergonal is recovered from the urine of post-menopausal

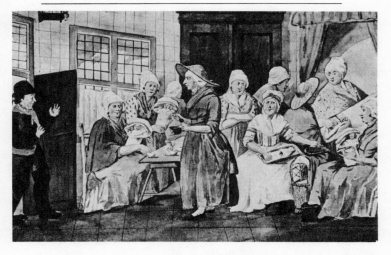

In 1719 quintuplets were born in a Dutch farmhouse. Note the midwives who hold the babies. Roads were black with carriages of people who came and paid a fee to see the babies. (Courtesy of the Bettmann Archive)

women and termed HMG or Human Menopausal Gonadotropin. Both hormones are FSH.

Procedure

The use of Pergonal is expensive and also presents a certain risk. This is why patients must be selected very carefully. All other causes of infertility must be ruled out, and the reason why the patient is anovulatory should be determined as closely as possible. The ovaries must be examined and the concentration of the sex hormones must be determined. Candidates for Pergonal therapy usually have low levels of estrogen, FSH, and LH.

The two major dangers of Pergonal therapy are multiple birth and the development of multiple ovarian cysts. In extreme cases the latter can rupture, and hemorrhage severely. This results in a medical emergency that can require the removal of the ovaries.

Since Gemzell first induced ovulation with FSH, physicians have learned to supervise their patients very carefully so as to gauge treatment daily. This is man's way of attempting to duplicate what nature does so easily.

If you are selected for Pergonal therapy because you do not menstruate, you will first receive a course of progesterone to cause you to bleed. Five days after progesterone withdrawal bleeding, you will receive a first dose of Pergonal by injection. From then on you will have to come to the doctor's office every day, even on Sundays and holidays.

The physician will palpate your ovaries by a pelvic examination to determine that they are not excessively swollen, and measure the estrogen level. Estrogen levels are gauged by testing the cervical mucus, looking at a vaginal smear, and by measuring the estrogen in the blood.

The proper dosage of Pergonal is redetermined every day and may be increased. Toward the end of the treatment you may receive as much as six ampules a day. When the level of estrogen corresponds to that attained just prior to ovulation in normal women (this takes anywhere from seven to eighteen days of therapy), Pergonal is discontinued, and human chorionic gonadotropin therapy instituted. If there is no increase in body temperature the next morning to confirm ovulation, you receive another injection of HCG.

Final proof as to whether you have ovulated will be supplied by the progesterone levels determined eight to ten days after the administration of HCG. An increased level of progesterone can only be due to the corpus luteum that has taken the place of the departed ovum, which by then has been either fertilized or disintegrated.

This recently developed elaborate monitoring of the estrogen level has reduced the number of multiple births. The rate is still high (20–45 percent of all Pergonal births), as is the number of spontaneous abortions.

Complications due to Pergonal therapy are identical with those discussed for HPG. Treatment with Pergonal is not only expensive, it is emotionally trying. The daily treatment with an unknown endpoint and unpredictable results will tax even the most stable and determined individuals.

It goes without saying that at present Pergonal therapy should be given only by physicians very skilled in its use. As with other techniques physicians are learning more and more about this rather novel medical tool, and it is probably fair to say that the use of fertility drugs will become safer and even more successful in years to come.

Prolactin Hormone

Some women who do not menstruate develop fluid in their breasts. The amount of fluid may be scant and produced only by pressure on the nipple, or the fluid may escape spontaneously in amounts sufficient to soil a bra. This condition is termed galactorrhea and is often associated with an increase in the production of the hormone prolactin by the pituitary gland.

The persistence of breast secretion and failure to menstruate for an indefinite period after childbirth has been labeled the Chiari-Frommel Syndrome. These symptoms may continue for the remainder of the woman's life. Spontaneous remissions have been reported. Ovulation has been induced in some patients by the use of clomiphene.

Galactorrhea and amenorrhea may also be the result of abnormal pituitary function or a pituitary tumor. When the condition is associated with increase in the prolactin hormone in the blood, the pituitary gland must be examined. This is accomplished by a special X-ray technique, termed tomography, which involves taking X-ray pictures at different levels within the skull. Even tiny tumors can be identified this way and removed relatively simply.

Recently a drug called Bromergocryptin has been developed that induces ovulation and menstruation. It reduces prolactin in the blood and restores ovulation and menstruation.

This drug is not used if a tumor exists. As it is still in an experimental stage it is not available in the United States at this time.

Women who do not menstruate should examine their breasts for telltale fluid and have a blood test for prolactin. If increased prolactin is present, the skull should be examined by tomography.

10

MORE ABOUT
HORMONAL
DISORDERS

*To me man is . . . packed with chemical factories; his every cell
a better chemist and physicist than all the Nobel laureates put
together . . .*

—Abraham Myerson

A FULL BEARD AND A HAIRY CHEST ARE CONSIDERED SIGNS OF MASCU-
linity and virility. Many a man is happy to display his hairy
chest at the beach or have it peek through a V-neck shirt.

In a woman hairiness is less treasured. Most women
equate clear unblemished skin with femininity. Women who
have "real" beards used to be considered circus attractions—
one paid a few cents to see the bearded lady at the country fair.

The numerous magazine advertisements extolling the vir-
tues of bleaches, and other methods, for the control or eradica-
tion of "unwanted hair" attest to the fact that a certain degree
of hairiness is both common and despised. For some women
unwanted body hair is quite an emotional burden. Such excess
body hair in a women is termed hirsutism.

Women, as well as men, produce male hormones, called
androgens, from two powerful little glands located on top of
each kidney. (These glands, the adrenals, produce about forty-
five different hormones.) The androgens produced by the adrenals play an important role in the formation of sexual hair—
that is facial, pubic, and under-arm hair.

The ovaries also make their own brand of androgen which, like the androgen produced by the adrenals, contributes to hair growth. Estrogen, one of the other major hormones produced by the ovaries, counteracts the effect of the androgens produced by the adrenals.

The human skin contains tiny follicles which, when properly stimulated by hormones, will grow hair. These follicles are present on all skin surfaces except the palms of the hand and the soles of the feet. Potentially both men and women could grow hair on any skin surface.

At puberty the hair follicles become stimulated by the increasing tide of sex hormones. Boys grow hair on their faces, in the pubic area, legs, chest, and in their armpits. In girls the response is much more limited. Many women nevertheless develop a certain degree of hairiness. This usually is a familial trait, particularly pronounced in women of Mediterranean origin.

Far from being excessively masculine, these women seem to be particularly sensitive to the androgens produced by the ovaries and adrenals. After hormonal malfunction has been ruled out, women who are unhappy about their unwanted hair are advised to seek out the services of a good electrologist.

Hirsutism can, in a small proportion of cases, also be a sign of infertility. When observed during the physical examination of an infertile woman, it must be carefully evaluated. You should report to your physician any measure—such as shaving, bleaching, depilation, or electrolysis—that you have taken to minimize or eliminate body hair. Not reporting such measures could make a diagnosis more difficult.

Women whose infertility or sterility is associated with hirsutism may have dark hair on their upper lip and chin. Their nipples might be ringed with hair and fuzz may appear on their chest, between the breasts. The pubic hair extends straight up to the navel, and may extend down over the upper thighs. Sometimes the hair growth is so vigorous that it has to be shaved daily during the bathing season.

Other telltale signs are pimples, oily skin, and acne. Little white streaks (stria) appear over the fatty portions of the lower abdomen and on the upper thighs.

Hirsutism by itself does not result in infertility. But it is a symptom of two disorders—both of which can be responsible for the patient's inability to bear children. Both conditions are related to hormonal inbalance, but before treatment is instituted, the physician must determine which hormone system —adrenal or pituitary—has malfunctioned.

Polycystic Ovaries

Forty years ago Drs. Stein and Leventhal of Chicago noted a previously unidentified ovarian defect in some of their patients. The principal feature of this disorder was irregular menstruation or outright failure of menstruation (amenorrhea). The patients often had hirsutism. In some cases they had poorly developed breasts and were obese. The ovaries of many of the patients were extremely large.

When looked at with a Decker culdoscope or a laparo-

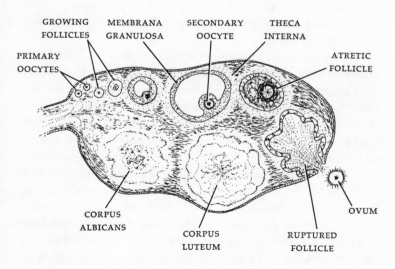

GROWING FOLLICLES   MEMBRANA GRANULOSA   SECONDARY OOCYTE   THECA INTERNA

PRIMARY OOCYTES   ATRETIC FOLLICLE

CORPUS ALBICANS   CORPUS LUTEUM   RUPTURED FOLLICLE   OVUM

Events that take place in a normally functioning ovary each month

scope, the ovaries seem studded with ova that had not ruptured, but instead turned into cysts. The condition was christened polycystic ovaries. It also goes by the name of the co-discoverers—the Stein-Leventhal Syndrome.

Drs. Stein and Leventhal found that in a large group of patients polycystic ovaries accounted for 4.3 percent of infertility.

After the hormones that govern ovulation became better understood, it was discovered that the Stein-Leventhal Syndrome is associated with gross abnormalities of the production of hormones by both the pituitary and the ovaries. Many patients suffering from polycystic ovaries also produce an excess of androgens, a fact that accounts for the hairiness. Today the syndrome is often diagnosed by determining the levels of various hormones in the blood or urine of the patient. The presence of polycystic ovaries should be confirmed by culdoscopy or laparoscopy.

During each menstrual cycle one or occasionally two or more of the primitive oocytes grow into a small cyst, called a follicle, which ruptures and expels the ovum.

In the polycystic ovarian syndrome the cyclic monthly development of the follicle fails, and the ovum remains in its follicle inside the ovary.

The frustrated pituitary continues to pour out FSH, which causes other follicles to develop. These also fail to complete their growth and do not expel their ova. Gradually many partially matured follicles become trapped in the ovary. The ovaries increase in size and sometimes become as large as a hen's egg. The ovaries also often become encapsulated by a tough membrane that further impedes the escape of a ripe ovum.

Once diagnosed, the Stein-Leventhal Syndrome should be treated even if the patient, for the moment, has no plans for becoming a mother. Uncorrected, the condition can result in masculinization, deepening of the voice, excessive facial and body hair, obesity, and enlargement of the clitoris. There also is some evidence that untreated women have a higher incidence of tumors of the uterus.

The preferred treatment at present is the cyclic administration of estrogen and progesterone, readily available as the birth control pill. Such treatment usually prevents the disease from progressing further because it suppresses the production of FSH, and hence the development of oocytes into ova that, in this instance, may become "stuck" in the ovary. The estrogen component of the birth control pills also inhibits the excess androgen production of the adrenals. When the pill is taken regularly, in a cyclic manner, the patient will have a monthly "withdrawal" bleeding akin to menstruation.

The administration of birth control pills, no matter what the purpose, prevents ovulation and thus pregnancy. The pills must be discontinued when a woman who suffers from polycystic ovarian disease wants to conceive. Her ovaries, however, may not be able to expel matured ova.

When Drs. Stein and Leventhal first discovered the condition, they found that it could often be treated by a very simple surgical operation called a "wedge" resection. During surgery a wedge-shaped piece is removed from the large ovary, permitting the eggs to be released from inside the capsule. The operation also results in a decrease in the size of the ovaries. This often causes a return to ovulation and menstruation, and actually improves fertility. Regular menstruation occurs in 80 percent of patients and a 60-percent pregnancy rate has been reported.

Today the Stein-Leventhal resection is seldom used. Instead the condition is now treated with clomiphene citrate—the anti-estrogen hormone discussed in the previous chapter. This drug stimulates the production of FSH, apparently providing the ovum with enough pep to leave the ovary. If clomiphene therapy fails, a wedge resection of the ovaries is resorted to.

Patients suffering from polycystic ovaries do not always exhibit the classic symptoms. Every infertility specialist can cite cases of women who came to the office complaining of infertility who were neither particularly hairy, nor obese, and some who even menstruated regularly. In one particular case polycystic ovaries were discovered by accident when the patient underwent a culdoscopic examination. In this instance the forty-one-year-old woman was successfully treated with both a wedge resection and fertility pills. She only needed one course of therapy and gave birth to healthy twin girls.

Adrenal Hyperplasia

The most characteristic features of polycystic ovarian disease—hirsutism, amenorrhea, and infertility—are shared with another condition: adrenal hyperplasia (the name implies overactive adrenals).

Before therapy is instituted for either polycystic ovarian disease or adrenal hyperplasia, one of the conditions must be carefully ruled out by differential diagnosis.

Since adrenal hyperplasia is not associated with enlarged ovaries, the presence of the latter may be used as a distinguishing feature. (Very large ovaries can be felt by a simple pelvic examination.) A simpler and more sure-fire method is a detailed hormone analysis of the blood and urine of the patient.

Adrenal hyperplasia is characterized by an excess amount of adrenal hormones, including androgens. It is usually treated with small doses of the hormone cortisone, which depresses the action of the adrenal glands and thus reduces the amount of hormones produced. If appropriate, cortisone therapy, continued over a period of several months, will restore menstrual regularity and improve fertility.

Correction of either the Stein-Leventhal Syndrome or adrenal hyperplasia will control the excess body hair growth.

In some cases the excess body hair will disappear following therapy. Hair that remains after the conditions have been brought under control can be removed by electrolysis.

Post-pill Amenorrhea

Another problem that has received increasing attention is the fact that some women stop ovulating—and menstruating—after they have discontinued oral contraceptives. Post-pill amenorrhea, as the condition is called, affects about one-half of 1 percent of all pill users. The failure to resume normal menstruation is not related to the length of time a person has been on the pill, nor is it a general phenomenon. The great majority of pill users resume normal menstruation within three months. Similarly, neither prior pregnancy nor childbearing protects a woman against developing the condition.

At present there is considerable speculation as to whether birth control pills do induce the amenorrhea, or whether the condition only occurs in women who are predisposed to irregular menses and ovulatory failure. Initial studies along these lines seem to bear out the second conclusion, and some specialists feel that women who have irregular periods should not use oral contraceptives at all.

Most women who suffer from post-pill amenorrhea and wish to conceive are at present treated with clomiphene. Bromergocryptin has also been used successfully on an experimental basis. (Both these drugs were discussed in Chapter 9.)

11

INFECTIONS AND
INFERTILITY

As it takes two to make a quarrel, so it takes two to make a disease, the microbe and its host.

—Charles V. Chapin

INFECTIOUS AGENTS PLAY A MAJOR ROLE IN MANY MEDICAL PROBLEMS—and infertility is no exception. In spite of the tremendous advances made in the control of infections, many infertility specialists feel that the problem is on the increase.

The reemergence of infections as an important concern in medicine is surprising, and a little ironic. Fifty years ago they were the major cause of death. A pelvic infection was a serious threat to life, as were pneumonia, tuberculosis, and childbed fever. Since there was no way to combat infections directly, the only effective measure was preventive. Strict adherence to asepsis during surgery, isolation wards, and other conservative measures reduced the number of fatalities.

The advent of sulfonamides, penicillin, and other antibiotics seemed to make all these prophylactic measures unnecessary. Many physicians then became rather cavalier about infections because one could always quell the disease swiftly with one of those marvelous products supplied by the pharmaceutical industry.

But now the "bugs" are striking back. As Dr. William J.

Ledger of the University of Southern California School of Medicine says: "We are relearning that bacteria can adapt to a hostile environment."

The infertility specialist is not concerned with acute infections but rather with the destruction caused by the microorganisms that manage to invade the genito-urinary tract or the peritoneal cavity. The damage wrought may only be discovered decades after the original infection has been brought under control. Often the primary infection has gone unnoticed.

The destruction that may be responsible for your inability to conceive is believed to result from irritation and inflammation of the tissues at the site of infection. The body, in the process of repairing the insult, may form scar tissue that can block or destroy the architecture of something as delicate as the Fallopian tubes or the cilia.

Sometimes two inflamed surfaces may become stuck together; sometimes the surfaces may pull apart after they have healed, but a few adhesions are left as a reminder of the infection. Such adhesions may block the tubes or entangle both tubes and cilia, preventing them from performing in a normal fashion.

Of all the infectious agents that can invade the genito-urinary tract or the peritoneal cavity, gonorrhea is the must troublesome as far as the infertility patient is concerned.

The availability of female methods of birth control, together with the generally more relaxed sexual mores of our times, contribute to the almost epidemic proportions of VD now seen at all levels of society. Gonorrhea is at present the leading cause of infertility among patients coming from lower economic groups. With the skyrocketing increase of VD among all segments of the population, but especially teenagers, it may become the dominant cause of infertility for all population groups in years to come.

Gonorrhea also is a prime example of a microorganism that adapts itself to existing medications. A few years after penicillin was introduced as a cure, some strains of gonococcus developed resistance to the then commonly used doses. In some patients, treated with what was then considered adequate therapy, the disease progressed. Furthermore, after the introduction of penicillin, physicians noted that there was a considerable increase in tubal pregnancy in patients who had had gonorrhea.

Apparently prompt treatment with antibiotics had prevented complete tubal closure but a partial narrowing of the tube had occurred. The oviduct was wide enough for the spermatozoa to pass in their upward track, yet the fertilized ovum could not make the trip back through the narrow channel and became stuck.

It is not generally known that gonorrhea can often exist in both sexes without overt symptoms. In the woman the organisms become lodged in the vagina and cervix. Often the only symptom is a slight vaginal discharge. The incidence of such subtle, insidious infections in women occurs in half of those exposed to gonorrhea.

If not recognized and treated, gonorrheal infections of the cervix have a 50 percent chance of eventually spreading to the Fallopian tubes. Here again the disease may be overlooked. The slight fever and minor lower abdominal discomfort are sometimes explained away as a "stomach virus," or a cold.

Usually, however, a patient whose gonorrhea spreads to the tubes will have fever and severe abdominal pain. The abdomen becomes extremely tender, and the routine pelvic examination is very painful. Technically the condition is classified as acute pelvic infectious disease—or p.i.d. for short—and its victims usually require immediate hospitalization. In most cases the acute inflammation subsides rapidly with antibiotic therapy.

Whether acute or subtle, gonorrhea that has spread into the peritoneal cavity often causes permanent alteration of the tubes, which in turn may cause infertility.

One of the oldest methods of birth control—the condom —has long been known to reduce the incidence of venereal disease. In ancient time condoms were made of cloth or animal gut. Gabriele Fallopius—the Italian anatomist who first described the oviducts or Fallopian tubes 400 years ago—initiated what was probably the first controlled study in medicine. At that time Italy and other parts of Europe were constantly plunged in armed strife. Armies and camp followers roamed the land, and venereal disease was rampant.

Fallopius discovered that the use of a linen sheath during intercourse prevented infection. The Italian doctor tested the sheath on 1,100 men and "called immortal God to witness" that none of them was infected.

Venereal disease is not the only infectious agent that contributes to the increase in pelvic inflammatory disease. Freely available abortion and other types of instrumentation involving the uterine cavity, such as the insertion of intrauterine devices, have all increased the risk of infectious disease and trauma.

In the past pulmonary tuberculosis often spread to the pelvic cavity, causing infertility. Today pelvic tuberculosis is rare in the United States.

Damage can also be caused by infections that originate in the pelvic cavity itself. Appendicitis even in childhood has often been implicated as a cause of infertility in women, because the disease is frequently associated with minor pelvic inflammatory disease.

Since pelvic inflammatory disease is on the increase, physicians now often test their infertility patients for infectious agents as a matter of routine. Special culture techniques can identify gonorrhea, as well as other types of vaginal and cervical infections.

A physician who discovers that his or her infertility patient has active disease will treat her with adequate medication for gonorrhea, tuberculosis, or whatever the case may be, and hope that the infection will subside without leaving a lasting mark. But this is often not the case.

Permanent damage, usually discovered long after the disease itself has subsided, must be repaired by appropriate means described in Chapter 12. In medicine an ounce of prevention is worth a pound of cure. Infections of any kind, but especially venereal, should receive prompt attention, and adequate methods of birth control—including the old barrier types such as the diaphragm and condom—are more desirable than an induced abortion.

Infections can also affect fertility in men. In addition to venereal disease and tuberculosis, which can cause infertility, mumps contacted after puberty can present a problem. The mumps virus can travel to the testes, causing intensive, acute inflammation (orchitis). Affected testicles—the condition can affect one testicle or both—become filled with fluid, which then presses on the delicate seminiferous tubules. It is this pressure, together with the virus itself, which may result in the permanent impairment.

Here, as in the case of other infections, it is best to treat the disease promptly during its active state by draining the accumulated fluid through a series of small incisions into the fluid sac. All physicians advocate adequate scrotal support during the active phase of the orchitis.

Orchitis is not necessarily a complication of mumps in adulthood, nor do all cases of orchitis result in infertility.

Mycoplasms

The infectious agents discussed so far cause alterations in the structure of the reproductive tract, which remain long after the disease has run its course. There is, however, another group of infectious agents that take up residence in the genital tract and are believed to interfere with conception or pregnancy.

Mycoplasms, as the organisms are now called, are still rather mysterious.

Until recently most mycoplasms have been implicated in some pulmonary infections, hence their former name—pleuripneumonia-like organisms, or PPLO for short. Only recently have two (T-mycoplasm and Mycoplasm hominus) been shown to play a role in infertility and habitual abortion.

They are microbial nudists, choosing to live without cell walls. Unlike viruses, which must live inside other cells, they can survive on their own.

Mycoplasms are very small, being intermediary in size

between viruses and bacteria. Under an ordinary light microscope they are not visible individually, but appear as colonies which look like a mass of branching filaments. In men they can cause a persistent inflammation of the prostate, and in women a chronic recurrent inflammations of the bladder and the endometrium.

Evidence for their role in infertility is that a particular form of T-mycoplasm has been isolated more frequently in infertile couples than in normal controls, and T-mycoplasms have been shown to cause infertility in domestic animals. Mycoplasm infections do not cause overt discomfort.

Exactly how mycoplasms interfere with conception or pregnancy is not yet known. Some investigators report that they have found mycoplasms actually attached to the sperm cells, suggesting that this might make forward progression of the sperm and fertilization more difficult. It has also been suggested that the organisms cause a sub-acute endometrial inflammation, which may interfere with the implantation process. Other suggestions are the possibility of a blighted ovum, infection of the embryo, destruction of the placenta, or various other minor changes that may lead to abortion.

All this is still rather doubtful. But adequate treatment of a diagnostically proven mycoplasm infection did improve fertility in 29 percent of couples with unexplained infertility. Infertility patients are not routinely tested for T-mycoplasm. The test is indicated when:

1—No other cause of infertility has been diagnosed.
2—The woman has had more than two spontaneous abortions, regardless of whether she previously carried her baby or babies to term.
3—Minimal sub-acute endometritis has been established by an endometrial biopsy.
4—There is a history of ectopic pregnancy.
5—The postcoital test is poor despite a normal sperm analysis.

Both partners should be tested for T-mycoplasm. In the man the test is done on a sperm sample obtained by masturbation and collected in a clean glass jar. In the woman the test is done on cervical mucus, preferably collected at midcycle.

In either case a small amount of specimen is placed in a small glass dish with a suitable culture medium. T-mycoplasms are finicky and their culture takes great care and experience. Evidence of growth appears after one or two days.

Treatment

If either culture is positive, the couple should be treated simultaneously because the organism can be transferred during intercourse. Condoms should be used until both partners are negative for T-mycoplasm.

Since T-mycoplasms do not have cell walls, they will not respond to ordinary antibiotics, which work because they prevent cell-wall formation. T-mycoplasms do respond to some potent antibiotics such as declomycin, monocyclin, and vibramycin.

If possible, the sensitivity of the organisms to the antibiotic should be determined before treatment is initiated. The test is done at the time of the first culture.

According to Dr. Masood A. Khatamee, Assistant Clinical Professor at New York University Medical School, in order to avoid the reemergence of the infection, it is important that both partners finish the prescribed course of treatment, which usually extends over ten days. Some of the antibiotics used cause such side effects as nausea, vomiting, and diarrhea. These symptoms will disappear, and treatment should if possible be completed.

Although the role of mycoplasms in infertility is not established beyond doubt, all patients with positive mycoplasm cultures should be treated until the cultures are negative.

12

ENDOMETRIOSIS

RECENTLY A LEADING DAILY NEWSPAPER CARRIED A NEWS ITEM HEAD-
lined: "Woman's Death Laid to a Rare Disease." The article
went on to describe the case of a twenty-two-year-old woman
who died as a result of massive internal bleeding. The medical
examiner's office was reported as saying that the hemorrhaging
was caused by a "very rare" ailment called endometriosis.

In fact the medical examiner was wrong. The reason that
he might have been unfamiliar with the disease is that it is rarely
if ever fatal. It is, however, very common, occurring more often
than appendicitis in ovulating women. It usually starts during
the childbearing years, and is a leading cause of infertility.

The disease at present remains one of the most puzzling
in gynecology. It was first observed in 1899. But it was only in
1920 that Dr. J. A. Sampson recognized its serious consequences and frequency of occurrence. In his now classic report
Dr. Sampson reported that during abdominal surgery in women
over thirty years of age, he occasionally noted that the pelvic
organs were stuck together as if glued. He also observed various
blobs and blisters filled with a dark, gummy material. In some

instances the tubes and ovaries were stuck to the uterus. Sometimes the uterus was twisted out of place and stuck to the rectum.

Dr. Sampson removed some of this gummy material and examined it under the microscope. It turned out to be old, clotted blood, which upon further examination contained cells normally found only in the lining of the uterus (endometrium). Identification of the nature of the cells partially solved the mystery. The curious disease was caused by endometrial cells that somehow had wandered from the uterus into the pelvic cavity. Hence the disease was called endometriosis. (The Greek ending *-osis* refers to an abnormal process.) Endometriosis is different from endometritis, which is an inflammation of the lining of the uterus.

The endometrium, like all other tissues of the body, consists of a collection of cells, which apparently can survive for a while after they become detached from the wall of the uterus.

Sometimes, for reasons still not understood, a few of these cells emigrate into the pelvic cavity. Dr. Sampson felt that this occurs at menstruation time, when some of the menstrual blood, containing endometrial cells, is regurgitated through the Fallopian tubes. Once they reach the pelvis they act almost like a skin graft, attaching themselves to various pelvic structures: the ovaries, the bowel, the outside of the uterus, the rectum, the bladder, and the delicate lining of the pelvis. Their final resting place seems to be purely a matter of chance.

Although the implants are tiny at first, they often manage to survive in their new environment. Soon a command to multiply and prepare for a fertilized ovum comes to the cells from the ovaries, transmitted via the hormones estrogen and progesterone.

The displaced endometrial cells respond just as if they were in the uterus. However, unlike their counterparts in the uterus, they are unable to separate and be cast off during the following menstrual period. The collection of cells sometimes bleeds a little. Once the menstrual cycle is over, the endometrial implants heal somewhat, only to be stimulated again during the next menstrual cycle.

The growing, healing, and bleeding cycles result in scarring and adhesions about the tubes, ovaries, and especially around the delicate tubal fimbria. Adhesions can also fix the ovary and tubes in a manner that interferes with the transfer of ova from the ovary to the tube.

The growing endometrial cells may invade the tough covering of the ovary. Once they dig in and multiply, they often collect large amounts of blood. This results in an ovarian blood cyst that can attain the size of a hen's egg or even an orange. With time the blood becomes dark brown, which is why these cysts are called chocolate cysts.

Endometriosis often is a cause of infertility, yet it is frequently overlooked. The senior author recalls a patient who came to see him with an infertility problem. Mrs. Barnes was twenty-six years old. While in college she had severe menstrual pains. She was put on oral contraceptives and her menstrual pain vanished almost immediately. She took the pill for four years, then she got married. In due time the young couple wanted to have children and the pill was discontinued.

After two unsuccessful years the prospective parents consulted a physician. Both the husband and the wife underwent routine testing for infertility and were told that all was normal. Time alone—it was said—would solve their problem. This evaluation was based on the fact that Mrs. Barnes ovulated regularly, and that her tubes were open when examined by a hysterosalpingogram (X-rays).

Eventually the couple consulted Dr. Decker, who became suspicious when Mrs. Barnes reported her past painful menstruations, which had returned after the birth control pill were discontinued.

He also noted that the patient was especially sensitive in one particular spot when he palpated the uterus. It was decided to examine the patient by culdoscopy. This procedure confirmed the presence of endometriosis.

Severe menstrual pains, sometimes beginning in the teens, often are suggestive of endometriosis. The condition can be overlooked because many people, including doctors, feel that discomfort during menstruation is a natural thing. Painful periods can—but need not—be a sign of endometriosis, but as the condition worsens periods become more uncomfortable. Endometriosis can also cause pain during intercourse.

Diagnosis is easy if the endometrial growths are extensive, because the masses have a characteristic lumpy consistency and are extremely tender to the touch. However, when the cysts are small and the discomfort negligible, diagnosis is not that simple since these symptoms are associated with a great variety of gynecological disorders.

Minor degrees of endometriosis, possibly responsible for infertility, can be spotted with a culdoscope or a laparoscope. Even the smallest bit of endometrial tissue can be seen upon examination with instruments that carry their own light source.

Treatment

Treatment depends on the degree of discomfort, the size of the endometrial growths, and the age of the patient.

Because the condition is clearly related to the cyclical hormonal stimulation associated with menstruation, and is suppressed during pregnancy (which often cures the condition permanently), treatment consists of inducing a state of pseudopregnancy. This is easily done today with birth control pills that contain both estrogen and progesterone. The procedure usually takes six to nine months. It will relieve many of the symptoms but normally does not prevent the adhesions and scarring left by the disease.

When endometriosis interferes with conception or pleasurable sexual intercourse, or is very extensive, or if the patient will subsequently want to become pregnant, it is usually advisable to remove as much of the endometrial tissue as possible by surgery. The surgeon must carefully cut out all endometrial growths, scar tissue, and adhesions on the ovaries, along the outside wall of the uterus, along the Fallopian tubes—or wherever else the endometrial cells have spread. Smaller growths are often destroyed by heat (cauterization). The surgery should be carried out with great care so as to enhance the patient's chances for pregnancy; if necessary the surgeon will also replace the reproductive organs in their normal position.

Surgery for endometriosis can, but need not be, extensive. The senior author has been able to remove small endometrial implants during exploratory culdoscopy.

Surgery for endometriosis is sometimes preceded by hormone therapy so as to shrink the endometrial tissue and soften the adhesions that surround the growths. Menstruation is suppressed with birth control pills both before and for a number of months after the operation.

Doctors generally agree that infertility problems in which endometriosis is the primary cause are more successfully treated with surgery than with hormonal therapy. In one study conducted by Drs. William Andrews and G. Douglas Larson of Norfolk, Virginia, the pregnancy rate in a group of women treated with drugs was 39 percent, as compared to the 59 percent noted in a group treated surgically.

Endometriosis can also be treated with male hormones that suppress the growth of endometrial tissue. These unfortunately have a masculinizing effect. Dr. Robert Friedlander, of the Medical College of the State University of New York, in Albany, reported an experience with Danazol, a new synthetic male hormone that apparently has a minimum of masculinizing side effects. Danazol has now been approved for general use.

As in the treatment with progestins and estrogen (birth control pills), Danazol is unable to dissolve the adhesions that have formed because of the endometriosis, or, for that matter, to replace the pelvic organs in a position more conducive to conception.

Endometriosis is rarely troublesome after menopause because the endometrial implants are no longer stimulated cyclically by sex hormones.

Infertility and Endometriosis

There is a distinct feeling among physicians that endometriosis is a modern disease, attributed to the current social climate that encourages late marriage and delays pregnancy. The malady is still uncommon in India and other societies where girls marry young and proceed to motherhood.

Indeed a very small chance of developing endometriosis exists during each menstrual cycle, when a few cells of the uterine lining may become detached and migrate in the wrong direction up the Fallopian tubes. The condition is probably on the increase because girls start to menstruate earlier in life than they used to. The average age of the menarche (onset of menstruation) in 1976 was twelve years and six months, as compared to fourteen years a century ago. Women thus experience many more menstrual cycles before getting around to motherhood, especially since the latter is also often postponed because of altered lifestyles. Furthermore the age of menopause is also increasing, prolonging the time a woman may be subject to the effects of the disease.

Other factors, no doubt, are at work. Gynecologists are in general agreement that the disease occurs more frequently in thin, intelligent, somewhat overactive women.

Not all women who are found to have endometriosis do have an infertility problem. Endometriosis is nevertheless a leading cause of infertility, sometimes accounting for up to 40 percent of the patients seen at a particular infertility clinic.

Endometriosis is a medical condition that is still best treated by surgery, especially if it causes an infertility problem. Even though it was first observed about eighty years ago, it remains almost a total mystery. Incidence figures are hard to come by, but it probably affects 10 percent of all women. Yet little research is devoted to uncovering its cause, to finding more conservative means of treatment, or ways of preventing its occurrence. Endometriosis is thus a good example of the current lack of scientific interest in much of reproductive biology.

13

SURGERY

No good physician quavers incantations
When the malady he's treating needs the knife.

—Sophocles

IT HAS OFTEN BEEN SAID THAT THE STATE OF CIVILIZATION OF A PARTICU-
lar society can be gauged from quality of the care that women
receive during childbirth. Operations to assist the mother during birth existed in antiquity. In pre-imperial Rome, in 700 B.C.,
there was even a law decreeing that an attempt should be made
to deliver a living child by opening the body of the mother
should she die during childbirth. It is said that Julius Caesar,
who forged the Roman Empire during the first century A.D., was
delivered in this manner. The operation has borne his name ever
since.

Surgical operations to help a woman conceive, or to help
her carry a baby to term, are of much more recent origin.

The type of surgical repair required will depend on the site
of the trouble. It goes without saying that a thorough diagnosis,
and perhaps even a consultation with another physician in case
major surgery is suggested, should precede any intervention.

Let us look once more at each of the structures involved
in reproduction, and determine how, if needed, they can be
repaired surgically.

The Cervix

The cervix, or neck of the uterus, gives some cause for concern from a surgical point of view. Under certain circumstances the muscles can be weak and the cervix will open prematurely (incompetent cervix). This can often be corrected by an operation called cerclage that is discussed in more detail in the chapter on miscarriage.

The cervical canal can also be partially or totally blocked (cervical stenosis). This condition may be inborn or it may be the result of injury, infection, or tumors.

Complete closure prevents menstrual bleeding. Partial closure becomes apparent when it is either impossible or difficult to pass a cannula through the cervical canal during a tubal insufflation test. The condition usually stems from recurrent cervical infections, previous surgery, biopsies, or other instrumentation of the cervix. At the time of examination the infection may be active, and the swelling can also partially block the cervix.

Local cervical infections may cause small growths (polyps) that once again can obstruct the cervical canal, and must be removed by surgery.

Extensive cervicitis is best treated by cryosurgery (*cryo* means cold). During cryosurgery the affected inflamed tissue is

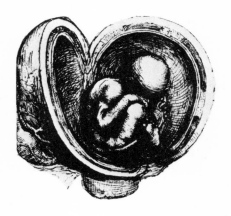

The great Italian artist, Leonardo da Vinci (1452–1519), was the first to show accurately the form of the womb. (Courtesy of the Bettmann Archive)

frozen to a very low temperature. The procedure is carried out in the doctor's office. Cryosurgery results in less scarring or constriction than conventional cauterization.

Some patients also have a congenitally small cervix that can be dilated in the office by careful stretching with an appropriate instrument.

The Uterus

The uterus often is a cause for reproductive failure. Its troubles can be divided into two major areas: malformations, and various benign growths. One possible but not invariable cause of infertility is uterine malformation. The uterus can be repaired surgically, but other factors that may be responsible for the infertility must be ruled out before such surgery is undertaken, because uterine malformations do not necessarily preclude pregnancy.

A study carried out at Johns Hopkins University School of Medicine by Drs. Howard W. Jones and Theodore A. Baramki shows that only one-quarter of women with a certain type of congenital abnormality fail to carry their babies to term.

The cause of uterine malformation is faulty or arrested embryonic development. Very early during embryonic life, at about week twelve, the sex organs begin to be formed. The very young embryo has both male and female internal genital ducts. One set, the Millerian ducts, have the potential to develop into Fallopian tubes, uterus, and portions of the vagina. The other tubal structure, termed the Wolffian ducts, develops into the vas deferens, seminal vesicles, and epididymis. The sex of the future child determines which of the embryonic structures will develop.

In the female the fusion of the ducts is incomplete at first, and the embryo has two separate cavities. Then the inner wall, or septum, that separates the cavities starts to degenerate. Eventually there remains a single cavity, the precursor of the uterogenital canal.

Sometimes this fusion is incomplete, in which case the

uterus of the grown woman will not assume its normal pear shape. If the embryonic fusion was a total failure, the patient may have two separate uteri of equal or unequal sizes. Sometimes only the upper border of the uterus remains deeply grooved and indented, and the uterus is heart-shaped. This deformity is known as a bicornate uterus.

All these malformations may reduce a woman's fertility. Uterine malformations are diagnosed by the special technique (hysterosalpingogram) detailed in Chapter 7.

Fibroids (Myomas)

Tumors of various kinds are very apt to develop in the uterus. If they are large, hemorrhage extensively, or are cancerous, they should be removed surgically. If the couple has had all the children they want, and the condition warrants it, it is simplest to remove the entire uterus by performing a hysterectomy (total excision of the uterus). Fortunately most tumors found in the uterus are harmless (benign) and today many surgeons are skilled at excising such growths by means of conservative surgery, salvaging the uterus itself so that the woman can still bear children. The operation is called myomectomy—removal of a myoma (the word "myoma" means growth of tumor consisting of muscle tissue). Myomas of the uterus are usually called fibroids because they contain fibrous tissue. Black women are particularly prone to develop fibroids.

Nobody quite knows how often infertility results from a fibroid tumor. As in the case of an abnormally shaped uterus, many women with fibroids of various sizes have conceived and carried to term without trouble. The size of the fibroid also is not necessarily related to the extent to which it may interfere with conception or implantation.

A small fibroid that blocks the entrance to the uterus either near the cervix or at the point of attachment of the Fallopian tubes may severely interfere with the migration of the sperm or ova; whereas the same size growth, located elsewhere in the uterus, may not. Some fibroids may interfere with the proper nutrition and function of the endometrium, and others may prevent the uterus from expanding sufficiently during pregnancy.

But none of this necessarily happens, and in patients in whom fibroid tumors are suspected to be the cause of infertility all other possibilities should be ruled out before a myomectomy is undertaken. Because fibroids may grow rapidly, women in whom the condition has been diagnosed should complete their families as swiftly as possible.

Much progress has recently been made in the treatment of all types of infertility, and myomectomies are no exception. Recent surveys made by several surgeons who performed operations on women whose infertility was strongly suspected to be caused by fibroid tumors indicated that about 25 to 50 percent conceived within two years after the operation. The number of spontaneous abortions occurring in women who underwent myomectomies is unfortunately much higher than in a normal control group.

Some surgeons perform repeat myomectomies on their patients. Drs. L. J. Malone and F. M. Ingersoll of the Massachusetts General Hospital in Boston report that several of their patients who failed to conceive after their first myomectomy had successful pregnancies after their second.

Dilatation and Curettage (D & C)

Before major surgery is undertaken, the patient sometimes first undergoes a small operation called dilatation and curettage—or D & C for short. The physician dilates the cervical canal and scrapes the sides of the uterus with a small spoon-shaped instrument called a curette. The material removed during this operation is then examined in a pathology laboratory. Small growths and adhesions may also be removed during the procedure, which may permit a couple to achieve the desired pregnancy.

Tubal Repair

One of the most common causes of infertility are the Fallopian tubes—the trumpet-shaped passages through which the ovum must travel from the ovaries to the uterus both before and after fertilization. Surgical repair of the Fallopian tubes is called tuboplasty.

The tubes are not simple conduits through which an egg rolls like a ball down a bowling alley. If they were, they might be more easily replaceable by some kind of substitute tubing. At one time or another surgeons have attempted to make oviducts out of the appendix, the ileum, arteries, or veins. Plastic tubing has also been tried. All these attempts have failed, but success may be around the corner. In 1975 Dr. Georg Sillo-Seidl, of the Paracelsus Clinic for Barren Couples in Frankfurt, Germany, transplanted Fallopian tubes, donated by women undergoing total hysterectomies, into three patients with partially occluded tubes. Although none of these women to date have become pregnant, the transplanted tubes were not rejected. Furthermore they appeared to be open and functional when examined by the standard tests.

One of the problems in replacing the tubes with tissue taken from elsewhere in the body is that on the inside the tubes are lined with cilia that push the egg along its path toward the uterus for implantation. The cilia magnified would look much like a wheat field waving in the wind.

The oviducts actively participate in the process of fertilization, somehow managing to accommodate two-way traffic—upward for the sperm and downward for the ovum both before and after fertilization. Special nutrient secretions in the lining of the tube are essential for the growth and nutrition of the fertilized ovum during its transport through the Fallopian tube.

To make matters more complicated, the tubes are convoluted and rather long, measuring about 4 1/2 inches.

At their upper or "distal" end, the tubes flare out into a series of projections—the fimbria, which act like minute fingers catching the ovum as if it were a ball. Once the ovum is caught,

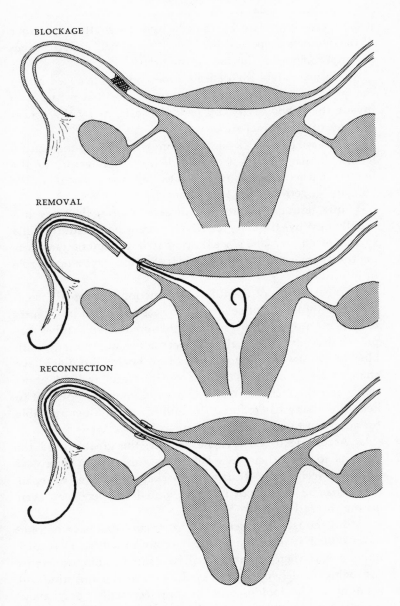

BLOCKAGE

REMOVAL

RECONNECTION

The Fallopian tubes are now repaired by surgeons with increasing success. Here the portion of the tube that is blocked is cut out. Then the tube is reconnected.

it is moved downward by the cilia and the rhythmic motions of the oviducts proper. At the lower, "proximal" end, the tubes are attached to the "horns" of the uterus.

Unfortunately the delicate tubes can be damaged rather easily by infectious or inflammatory disease that manages to invade the pelvic cavity, by endometriosis, or by the consequences of abdominal surgery.

Disease may block the tubes anywhere along their entire length. It may also destroy the delicate architecture of the fimbria that retrieve the ovum, coalescing two or several of the "fingers" together in an amorphous lump.

Infectious or inflammatory disease affecting the tubes also usually destroys the cilia, for which there is no substitute. Cilia seldom regenerate, and since they are so important in transporting the ovum to its destination, their absence plays a major role in infertility.

Whether or not the tubes are functioning properly is established by means of several of the tests detailed in Chapter 8. Until recently surgeons seldom attempted to repair tubes that proved defective. When all tests were done, most patients with blocked tubes were told to go and adopt a baby. But times have changed. Better methods of birth control, freely available abortions, and the fact that many unmarried mothers now opt to keep their baby has reduced the number of children available for adoption to a trickle.

According to Dr. Wayne Decker, the greater need for patients to have their own babies has resulted in improved operative techniques. Today Dr. Decker undertakes to repair tubes that he would not have attempted to operate on even during the early 1970s.

But though Dr. Decker and other surgeons have become more skilled at repairing tubes, they are unwilling to predict how many of their operations will be a success. (Success in this case being the delivery of a live baby.) Often the operation will result in healthy-looking tubes but not necessarily a pregnancy.

Tubal repair remains a difficult operation and the outcome is chancy. Dr. Decker usually tells his patients that without it their chance of conception is one in a million. Surgery, if performed by a skilled physician, will give the patient a "reasonable chance" (figures of success vary from 20 to 70 percent).

Anyone contemplating tuboplasty will have undergone extensive diagnostic tests. Most physicians will also attempt to open their patients' tubes by conservative measures such as repeated injection of the tubes with corticosteroids and antibiotics (hydrotubation).

Candidates for tubal repair should be further evaluated by culdoscopic or laparoscopic examination. Those selected for surgery on the basis of defects identified by direct inspection have a better chance for success than patients in whom such a careful examination has been omitted.

Patients whose infertility problem is caused by tubal occlusion usually need both tubes repaired, because disease often affects both oviducts. Women with one functioning tube often conceive and so do not show up at an infertility clinic.

Since the Fallopian tubes are about 4 1/2 inches long, the repair may involve one of several techniques, depending on the nature and location of the trouble. Tubal surgery has been broken down into the following four areas:

Salpingolysis: Removal of adhesions around the tubes.
Salpingoplasty: Refers to repair of the opening (fimbrioplasty) of the closed tube, which involves the distal end of the tube and repair of the fimbria.
Uterotubal implantation: Removal of closed portion of the tube and replacing the end into the uterus.
Midsection reconstruction: Required when the tubes were tied, and the patient wants them reopened.

Salpingolysis

The simplest type of surgery involving the tubes is the removal of adhesions that cling to the oviduct from the outside—like vines to a drainage pipe. In the case of the soft oviducts such adhesions may easily interfere with the passage of the sperm and egg. The tubes can also become strangled by endometrial growths. Adhesions between the tubes and other pelvic organs such as the bowel or the ovaries may hold the tubes in a kinked position, which interferes with the normal pattern of traffic. Such conditions occur rather frequently. About 35 percent of all operations carried out to correct infertility problems involve salpingolysis.

The surgery involved in the repairwork can be minor (small adhesions or endometrial tissue can be removed during a culdoscopic or laparoscopic examination) or can involve major surgery. Whether minor or major, the operation should be carried out in the most gentle manner possible because otherwise new adhesions, resulting from fresh trauma, may replace those that have been so carefully removed. Good postoperative care is important with this as well as with any other type of tubal surgery.

Salpingolysis is a rather successful operation. On the average 40 percent of patients undergoing the procedure conceive and carry their babies to term.

Salpingoplasty

The first recorded surgical attempt at repairing diseased fimbria was made in 1881 by a German surgeon who operated on a twenty-one-year-old woman. Unfortunately he failed to report whether or not his patient conceived; chances are that she did not. In 1891 a Dr. Martin reported a series of twenty-four cases, but only one patient became pregnant and then had a spontaneous abortion. For a while thereafter surgeons simply removed the entire diseased fimbrial end of the tubes—not surprisingly no pregnancies resulted. Only later did it become known that the fimbria are essential to the reception of the ovum.

Today surgeons often attempt to tease the fimbria apart with as little destruction as possible. If the oviduct is closed at the upper end, an opening is made and a plastic tubing inserted to keep the area open. This tubing is placed so that it can be removed without surgery. Some surgeons prefer to protect the fimbria end of a tube that has just been operated on with a little silastic (a kind of plastic) hood. These plastic hoods have to be removed in a second abdominal operation. Other types of fimbrial prosthesis are in the process of being developed.

Good operative results are obtained if the fimbria are not too damaged. Results are still poor when the defects are extensive.

The operative procedure is followed by regular postoperative tubal lavage (hydrotubation) with corticosteroids and antibiotics. This prevents inflammation and infection, both of which could cause renewed damage.

Utero-tubal Implantation

If the blockage is in the vicinity of the point where the tubes are attached to the uterus, the surgeon severs the connection, removes the diseased portion of the tube, and reimplants the tubes into the uterus.

This type of blockage often results from venereal disease, especially gonorrhea, and the condition has been on the increase in all socioeconomic groups during the past decade. The condition can also result from a number of other factors, such as endometriosis, congenital malformations, a previous pregnancy, or complications arising from abortion, whether spontaneous or induced. Utero-tubal implantations account for 20 percent of all tubal repairwork.

The success of the operation again depends on the extent of the disease. But the success level rose considerably when surgeons started to insert the small plastic splints described earlier.

Once again postoperative care is very important. Much

benefit is derived from the administration of corticosteroids (before, during, and after surgery), which improve healing. Antibiotics are also given routinely because it has been observed that surgery often reactivates chronic tubal inflammatory disease. Finally many surgeons feel that a course of hydrotubation instituted after the plastic splints have been removed is most effective.

Rates of success for the operation vary considerably—the best being about 30 percent.

Midsection Reconstruction

This operation is most often required to undo a voluntary sterilization, so the details are discussed in the section devoted to that subject (Chapter 20). Success rates are still relatively low but will undoubtedly increase in the near future.

Ectopic (Misplaced) Pregnancy

Any pregnancy that occurs outside the uterus itself is called an ectopic pregnancy. Most such pregnancies occur in the Fallopian tubes. Very rarely an ovum is fertilized by an overeager sperm before it is expelled from the ovarian follicle. In this latter case one speaks of an ovarian pregnancy. Sometimes the fertilized ovum migrates into the pelvic cavity.

Though an ectopic pregnancy is proof of ovulation, fully open tubes, and the fact that the husband is fertile, it offers little cause for comfort. An embryo growing in the wrong place will rarely develop to full term.

Until recent times the condition was fatal in the great majority of cases because the almost inevitable rupture of the Fallopian tubes is accompanied by severe hemorrhaging. For a long time a pregnancy occurring outside the uterus was believed to be the consequence of violent emotions that accompanied conception. A typical story was that it occurred in women surprised in the arms of their lovers by their husbands.

By the middle of the nineteenth century physicians

started to suspect that ectopic pregnancies were the consequence of pelvic inflammatory disease, or that they were caused
by some malfunctioning of the Fallopian tubes.

Today it is known that an ectopic pregnancy is usually
caused by a minor defect of the Fallopian tube. The tiny sperm
can move upward through the narrowed tube, but the voyage
of the larger ovum to the uterus may be more difficult.

The whole event can be compared to the small boy who
puts his hand into a candy jar. His empty hand can fit through
the neck of the bottle, but the fistful of candy cannot be extracted that easily.

The fertilized ovum may also get stuck at a narrow point
of the Fallopian tube. It nevertheless continues to grow. The
special feeders (trophoblasts) dig into the lining of the tube to
gather nourishment for the embryo, just as if it had reached the
uterus.

The embryo continues to grow. It distends the tube until
the latter cannot stretch any further.

What happens next depends on the location of the pregnancy in the tube. If the point of attachment is near the fimbrial
end of the tube, the embryo may be pushed out (aborted) into
the abdominal cavity. Pregnancies located midway in the Fallopian tube usually rupture the oviduct. In either case there is
internal bleeding, various degrees of shock, acute pain, and the
possibility of death.

At best a tubal pregnancy usually causes permanent damage, or even the total loss of a Fallopian tube.

The problem is of special concern to the infertility specialist because the chances of a second ectopic pregnancy occurring
in the same tube are extremely high. Only 20 to 30 percent of
women who have had a tubal pregnancy are thereafter able to
achieve a successful one.

There is little that can be done at present to prevent a
tubal pregnancy, but it is most important to diagnose it before
it causes hemorrhage or other serious damage. In high-risk patients either laparoscopic or culdoscopic examination is carried
out when there is a suspicion of ectopic pregnancy.

Ectopic pregnancy occurs when some minor defect in the tubal lumen does not permit the fertilized ovum to reach the uterus. Most patients who have an ectopic pregnancy have experienced a period of infertility. The missed period that suggests pregnancy may be followed by scant bleeding. The pelvic examination will reveal a very tender tube. The pregnancy test may not be positive. The pregnancy may develop to six weeks before giving serious symptoms. There may be a sudden onset of severe pain in the lower abdomen. Pain and internal bleeding may cause fainting.

The chances of salvaging a tube have improved greatly since gynecologists have started to use microsurgical techniques, borrowed from eye and blood vessel surgery. Small instruments such as forceps and fine suturing material are used throughout the procedure, which is sometimes carried out under a magnifying glass.

It is believed that this technique inflicts less trauma on the tube, and results in less scar tissue to interfere with subsequent pregnancies.

Surgery in every field is becoming increasingly successful. Infertility patients can expect to profit from new developments in the years to come.

14

MISCARRIAGE

"It takes nine months to make bread," said the elder Murica.
"Nine months?" asked the mother.
"The grain is sown in November and harvested in July."
The old man counted the months: "November, December,
January, February, March, April, May, June, July. Just nine
months. It also takes nine months for the wine to mature; from
March to November. . . . That makes nine months too."
"Nine months?" asked the mother. She had never
thought of it before. The same length of time it takes to make a
man.

—Ignazio Silone, *Bread and Wine*

DIANA AND HANK M. HAD JUST BEEN MARRIED. SHE WAS BARELY TWENTY
and he twenty-two, about to be drafted into the Army for
service in Vietnam. Since a baby would keep him from overseas
duty, they opted for immediate parenthood.

For Diana this was an easy decision. When anyone had
asked her as a child what she wanted to be, she had always
answered: "A mother." Her feelings about motherhood did not
change when she majored in voice. Her main career goal, as she
recalled, was to be able to sing lullabies to her children. Since
she herself was an only child, she hoped to produce a houseful
of tots.

It took Diana six months to conceive. By that time Hank
was in the Army, and they were stationed in a camp in California. Every woman in sight was pregnant.

"The Army was the place to have your children," Diana
recalled years later. "They were practically free."

Diana enjoyed her pregnancy. "I felt very special. I could
hardly wait to buy my first maternity blouse. I even felt that it

was a privilege for Hank to hold my arm."

The bliss was not to last. One night Diana woke up with terrible cramps. She went to the toilet and passed, as she described it, "a big, bloody mess, my child."

Diana tried again and conceived after another six months. Her confidence had been shaken somewhat. She looked at all the other pregnant women on the base with somewhat mixed feelings and wondered whether they were better equipped than she to carry a child. They might have been, for Diana miscarried again during her first trimester (three months) of pregnancy.

When she conceived for the third time, and special tests indicated that her progesterone level was low, the Army doctor put her on Delalutin, a form of progesterone. Diana seemed to be doing fine.

Since life at the Army base was hectic, she decided to move in with Papa and Mama where life for her and her forthcoming baby would be quiet and uneventful. She selected a competent private physician, who looked at her medical records and decided that the Delalutin was superfluous. He discontinued the shots, and one Friday Diana noticed the by then familiar cramps.

Diana ended up in the emergency room of the local hospital and underwent another D & C.

Hank's turn in the Army ran its course, and when he came home they continued to try. Most of the joy had gone out of their marriage. As Diana recalls, "I had become totally obsessed with attempting to become a mother. I knew that it was my fault, I felt guilty, and I took it out on Hank. He was much more level-headed about it all. 'Yes,' he said, 'it would be nice if we had children, but if we don't we'll make other arrangements.'

"I could not see it that way. I kept hoping and going to the doctor, even though by then I had lost all faith in the medical profession.

"People told me to go and take a job, but I couldn't. I knew they thought that I was lazy. But I wasn't—I simply did not have the emotional strength to work. Besides I had to go to the doctor, and that had become a full-time occupation.

"I started doing crazy things, like poking my breasts to feel if they had become tender. I also had to go to the bathroom constantly to see whether 'the curse' had arrived.

"By then I was seeing a doctor who specialized in psychological infertility. I was getting both Clomid and Pergonal. I knew from my temperature chart that I was ovulating. With all the drugs I was taking I could have had seventeen children every month, but I did not conceive.

"Our medical bills were horrendous. We paid the doctors twice as much as we paid in rent, and still nothing happened.

"Throughout it all I felt totally alone.

"Fortunately I realized that I was in a state of total hysteria. I had nowhere to turn. I realized that I needed some kind of psychotherapy, and luckily I was able to afford the services of a psychiatrist.

"I went twice a week, and gradually I looked at miscarriage in a more realistic perspective.

"I still wanted children, but I was able to face the fact that Hank and I would never be natural parents. We would attempt to adopt. If that were to fail, we would try to find another way of putting our life back together. In the meantime I would go out and get a job.

"Well, maybe by that time I really had become psychologically infertile. A few months after I had resigned myself to that fate, I became pregnant.

"By then I had become a well-educated patient. I went to my gynecologist and insisted that he give me Delalutin. I carried my child to full term.

"The pregnancy was terrible. I always had had a tendency to have morning sickness, and the drugs I was getting made it worse. Often I could not keep any food down. I am not a very large woman, normally weighing only 100 pounds, but during pregnancy I only weighed 84 pounds!

"At one point my doctor gave me medication to control the morning sickness, but that misfired totally and I ended up in the hospital again where they fed me intravenously.

"Eventually my dream came true, and I gave birth to a

baby boy. Two years later we had a little girl. We are a very happy family now. Our kids are very special. Everybody says so, not only us. Hank is a particularly good father. Nevertheless I still cannot quite forget all the pain and anguish I went through, and I want to help others who might feel equally lost and unhappy."

Diana's problem is not rare. In the United States 10 percent of all pregnancies terminate spontaneously before the child is viable. Pregnancies that terminate before the fetus becomes viable (twenty-two weeks) are termed abortions. After twenty-two weeks they are termed miscarriages. "Stillbirth" implies the absence of life at birth of a viable fetus.

When an abortion occurs so early that the woman herself was not aware of the fact that she was pregnant, it is often referred to as a "silent abortion," and appears as a delayed menstruation. Women who miscarry after this initial period are often treated by the obstetrician whom they had chosen to deliver their baby.

Most abortions occur between the sixth and the tenth week of pregnancy. Women who experience more than two spontaneous abortions are classified as habitual aborters.

Women who aborted their first pregnancy have a 20 percent chance of losing their second.

Women who have given birth to one child and abort their second pregnancy are better off so far as the chance of successful future childbearing is concerned.

There are probably as many myths about how to avoid a miscarriage as there are about how *not* to become pregnant. Expectant mothers are cautioned not to hang curtains, nor to buy anything for the baby before it is actually born.

Until recent times doctors were almost as poorly equipped as the medicine man in helping patients who miscarried regularly. Their most common treatment was putting women to bed, but scientific studies have since proved that physical stress and exertion play a minor role in miscarriage.

The question of bed rest was tested by Dr. Edward C. Mann, director of the Recurrent Miscarriage Clinic of New

York Hospital. Dr. Mann divided his clinic population in two groups. Half of the women who started to stain, or experience mild cramps, were put to bed; the other half were allowed to continue with their normal daily routine, and merely asked to avoid overexertion. The number of miscarriages that occurred in either group was comparable, demonstrating that bed rest had no effect on the outcome of pregnancy.

The near-impossibility of dislodging a securely implanted fetus by physical means—such as falls, flagellation, prolonged horse rides, and comparable desperate measures—had also been amply proven by the many women who, throughout history, failed to rid themselves of an undesired pregnancy.

Causes of Abortion

Roughly speaking the causes of abortion can be divided into three categories:

1—A defective fetus
2—Faulty implantation of the fertilized ovum in the uterus, or other physical difficulty associated with the uterus or cervix
3—Hormonal deficiencies

Defective Fetus

Dr. George Streeter, of the Carnegie Institute of Embryology, in Washington, D.C., who spent most of his professional life studying the fertilized ovum and young embryo during the first days and weeks of its existence, often started his lectures by shelling a few pea pods. Chances were good, he said, that he would find a number of bad, runted peas.

Defective seeds are common among living creatures, and man is no exception. Figures are hard to come by, but it is estimated that about one-quarter of all unselected aborted feti were abnormal.

Abnormalities incompatible with the survival of the fetus

most often are due to "bad genes." Such a genetic defect can be contributed by either sperm or ovum. They can also result from an accident that occurred when the twenty-three chromosomes contributed by the mother combined with the same number contributed by the father. One of the twenty-three combinations may have been misplaced.

Sometimes the damage to the unborn results from disease suffered by the mother, usually during the first three months of pregnancy. Surprisingly, illnesses that can damage the fetus are often so mild that the mother was not even aware that she was ill, while a serious disease like cancer, or tuberculosis, does not hurt the fetus.

Several birth defects, such as mongolism, Tay-Sachs Disease, and Huntington's chorea, are caused by chromosomal abnormalities. Fortunately only 2 out of every 100 abnormal embryos develop to maturity; 98 percent are aborted before the end of the fourth month.

Sometimes—though extremely rarely—the embryo is adversely affected by a drug the mother has taken while she was pregnant. An innocuous sleeping pill, Thalidomide, caused phocomelia—a severe and rare birth defect characterized by partially missing limbs—in several thousand European children whose mothers had taken the drug during the early months of pregnancy.

The United States was spared this tragedy because the drug had not been cleared by the United States Food and Drug Administration. The United States, however, did not escape the ravages caused by the 1964–65 German measles epidemic. There was an increase in the number of spontaneous abortions. Many babies whose mothers had German measles during the first trimester of pregnancy suffered from various birth defects, including hearing loss, impaired vision, and heart disease.

Bad luck often is a hard taskmaster. The Thalidomide tragedy of the 1950s taught everybody a lesson, and today most drugs are tested for their birth defect–inducing capacity (teratogenicity) in animals. Physicians also prescribe drugs sparingly for their pregnant patients. The German measles experience has resulted in a widespread vaccination program for women who plan to become pregnant, though they must avoid pregnancy for a period of at least three months after immunization. Those who contract the disease in early pregnancy can choose to have a therapeutic abortion.

Finally, prospective parents who believe that their offspring may have a genetic defect—either because an earlier child is so affected or because the disease "runs in the family" —can avail themselves of a procedure called amniocentesis, which is described more fully in Chapter 18.

Very little can, or should, be done to prevent miscarriages that occur because the fetus was not viable. Though the grief of losing a hoped-for baby is intense at first, this is nature's way of safeguarding the health of the human race—or as Charles Darwin put it, assuring the "survival of the fittest."

Defects in Implantation (Nidation)

If you enjoy walking in the woods you occasionally will notice a fledgling tree growing in a spot that precludes its ever becoming a giant of the forest. The wind may have chosen to blow the seed into some soil collected on top of a rock, or among the roots of a much bigger tree. Geared to attempt survival at all cost, like all living things, the seed will sprout and send out some roots; but its stay on earth will be short.

A fertilized ovum has a much better chance of nesting itself securely and properly into the uterus than a wind-blown seed, and yet many a potential human being fails to nidate properly (nidation—derived from the French word for nest, *nid* —is the technical term for implantation).

Sometimes the fertilized ovum does not even manage to reach the uterus and starts growing in the tubes (ectopic pregnancy) or even in the peritoneal cavity. Most often a fertilized ovum reaches the uterine cavity. This journey normally takes five days. During this time the single fertilized egg cell grows and divides, into two, four, eight, and so forth cells. Each successive division doubles the number of cells. Soon a mass is produced that resembles a mulberry.

By the time it reaches the uterus it has become a hollow ball with small projections on its surface. It is now called a blastocyst. The projections on its surface are called trophoblasts —"tropho" meaning feeder or nourisher. Like the roots of the young tree that dig into the earth, the trophoblasts dig into the endometrium and start carrying nourishment from the mother to her developing young.

During these early days of pregnancy the blastocyst continues to change rapidly. By the time it is twelve days old, it has grown to measure nearly 1 millimeter. The trophoblasts continue to multiply and the placenta, which will take over the nourishment of the embryo, starts to form.

And yet the mother is not even aware of her pregnancy, because she is only about to miss her first period.

Mishaps are frequent during the complicated process of implantation and many a miscarriage occurs without anybody ever knowing that a possible future member of the human race was struggling for survival. This is why such very early miscarriages are called silent abortions.

The blastocyst continues to grow. Once it consists of more than one type of cell it is called an embryo. By the time it is thirty-two days old it measures 6 to 7 millimeters.

If the baby has been planned or hoped for, happiness settles in the home. Family and friends are informed, and the future mother is treated with special care.

Yet neither she nor her child is yet "home free." The manner in which the blastocyst has anchored itself to the wall of the uterus is crucial to the outcome of the pregnancy. If the place of implantation is favorable, such as the back wall of the uterus, near the top, all is well. If the blastocyst landed in the lower part of the uterus, near the cervix, there can be trouble because, in the course of pregnancy, the placenta may become detached and the woman expel the fetus prematurely.

An oddly shaped uterus may make nidation more difficult, and nonmalignant, fibroid tumors may make implantation difficult or impossible.

A fibroid, however, need not prevent implantation or cause a miscarriage. Every obstetrician will tell you of patients who conceive and give birth to a healthy child in spite of a large fibroid tumor, or an oddly shaped bicornate uterus. Malformed uteri, or fibroids that interfere with conception or cause repeated miscarriages, can be treated surgically (see Chapter 13).

Incompetent Cervix

The cervix, or mouth of the uterus, can be an unexpected source of trouble. The normal function of the cervix is to seal off the womb during the nine months of pregnancy, and open—wide —during labor. To accomplish this feat the cervix consists of ringlike muscles that normally are firm and tightly contracted. During pregnancy the cervix develops and stretches so as to accommodate the growing fetus. The muscles may, however, become weakened as a result of surgical operation—such as induced abortion—or previous labor. The cervix may also be maldeveloped congenitally. Whatever the cause, the cervix may start to dilate because of the pressure exerted by the increasingly heavy uterus. At one point the baby just falls out. If this occurs before the twenty-eighth week of pregnancy, the baby will fail to survive.

An incompetent cervix, as the condition is referred to, can now fortunately be corrected by simple surgical procedure. Women who have had repeated late abortions, or premature labors, should be examined frequently during the early months of pregnancy. The condition of the cervix is carefully observed at those times. If the cervix is incompetent, the fetal sac— commonly referred to as the "bag of water"—will be seen bulging through the gaping mouth of the uterus.

If indicated, the physician will reinforce the muscles with surgical suture material wrapped around the cervix as if it were a purse string. It is left in place during the remainder of the pregnancy. The operation is called cerclage, and refers to the fact that the cervix is held in place by a band or circle. The suture will not disturb the growing baby. It is easily removed at delivery, or shortly beforehand. Sometimes the doctor may recommend that the baby be delivered by Caesarean section. The suture must also be removed promptly if the patient goes into labor, because otherwise she might rupture her uterus.

Hormonal Deficiencies

It will come as no surprise to the attentive reader that some silent or habitual abortions are caused by a disturbance in the production of the hormones that play such an important role in the reproductive life of a woman.

During pregnancy, progesterone produced during half of each menstrual cycle by a temporary hormone production plant, the corpus luteum, plays a crucial role. It has been known since 1907, long before the hormones themselves were identified, that the corpus luteum is absolutely essential for the maintenance of the fertilized egg in the uterus. Indeed, accidental removal of the corpus luteum during the first ten weeks of pregnancy results in spontaneous abortion.

Thereafter—and this knowledge is derived from emergency abdominal surgery performed on pregnant women—the corpus luteum shrivels up as it does in a nonpregnant woman during menstruation. This finding indicates that after the tenth week of pregnancy the fetus can either do without progesterone, or this hormone is produced elsewhere.

Analysis of the urine of pregnant women ruled out the first possibility. In fact the concentration of pregnanediol (the breakdown product of progesterone found in the urine), which is an accurate reflection of the progesterone produced by the body, increases gradually from 4–10 mg. a day during the early weeks of pregnancy, to 70–80 mg. per day from the tenth week on.

A little more sleuthing demonstrated that the placenta takes over as the major—and eventually the only—progesterone production site during most of pregnancy.

The discovery that pregnancy urine contains much larger than normal amounts of pregnanediol—and estriol (the breakdown product of estrogen) proved crucial to those scientists who were attempting to isolate the twin hormones that govern reproduction in women. Science, however, always grows in more than one direction. The amount of progesterone present in pregnancy urine was of great interest to those who believed that a lack of progesterone might be responsible for a large fraction of the repeated or spontaneous miscarriages.

Urine analysis of women with characteristic signs of an incipient miscarriage (staining and cramps) showed that many of these patients had comparatively less pregnanediol in their urine than women who sailed through their pregnancy with flying colors.

This difference became particularly marked at about week eight, when progesterone production shifted from the corpus luteum to the placenta. The researchers speculated that in habitual aborters the placenta did not take over production at the right time.

In principle it should have been easy to determine whether the administration of progesterone did help certain selected patients carry their babies to term; but progesterone was practically unavailable in the late 1930s when scientists first asked themselves these questions.

Preliminary experiments carried out with progesterone—painstakingly extracted and purified from the urine of healthy women—seemed to so indicate. Gynecologists and their desperate patients kept clamoring for more hormone.

Finally Russell Marker, an organic chemist, abolished the progesterone famine by manufacturing progesterone from the roots of the Babasco plant found in Mexico. Not only did Marker's progesterone provide enough hormone to save the unborn, but by then it had been shown that it could also be used for birth control.

Since they were first developed in the 1950s, the various synthetic progestins that are the main components of the birth control pill have been taken by millions of women for contraception, acne, numerous menstrual disorders, endometriosis, and by selected patients during pregnancy.

Recently the enthusiasm for the indiscriminate use of these medications has decreased. It has been shown, for instance, that the offspring of women who were given certain progestins during pregnancy have a slightly higher incidence of congenital malformations, including heart defects. A female fetus may develop abnormal genitals. The question of whether to treat habitual aborters with hormones or hormone substitutes is thus at present a controversial one.

It is the feeling of scientists working closely with this problem that natural progesterones, whose use has not been associated with any increased incidence of congenital defects, may safely be used for women with abnormally low levels of progesterone.

Patients whose previous history indicates that their repeated miscarriages are associated with inadequate production of progesterone are subjected to exacting tests, during which the blood and urine level of progesterone and human chorionic gonadotropin are analyzed.

If the patient is pregnant, as indicated by the presence of human chorionic gonadotropic hormone, the blood progesterone level is determined. As soon as the level of progesterone is lower than normal, progesterone treatment is instituted. Delalutin, a natural progesterone, is given by injection or by vaginal suppositories. Progesterone is sometimes continued to about the twelfth week of pregnancy—or later if indicated by specific tests.

Progesterone bloodlevels are checked occasionally during treatment to make sure that they are within normal limits. Treatment of habitual abortion is successful in 60 percent of the cases.

The major difficulty is that treatment often is instituted too late to save pregnancy. The progesterone level will, however, prevent the expulsion of the fetus. Such "missed abortions" must then be terminated surgically by a D & C.

Psychological Factors

There is some evidence to indicate that severe or continual stress may be responsible for a few miscarriages. Some physicians have expressed the opinion that many women who habitually abort may be identified by their distinctive personality. The main factor is supposed to be an unwarranted fear that is neither expressed, suggested, or even hinted at by the patient. Severe emotional disturbances may trigger the uterus to extreme irritability or premature contractions that interrupt the pregnancy.

Like other psychological factors that may play a role in infertility, the facts for such an assumption are difficult to establish, and the many other possibilities that may cause an abortion should be ruled out before emotional factors are implicated.

Miscarriages, no matter what their cause, are hard to bear from an emotional point of view.

As illustrated by the history of Diana H., a purely physiological defect may become aggravated by psychological stress. It is important that both the physiological and psychological factors of a particular medical problem are adequately treated.

When asked whether she had any message for other women who may suffer from repeated habitual abortion, Diana said: "I would tell them to become very well educated patients. Looking back on my experience, I am ashamed to admit how little I knew about my own body, when I first started. I did not even know that women have fertile days!"

FOUR

COMMON
PROBLEMS

15

TROUBLE IN THE BEDROOM

Mix equal amounts of damask rose petals, gilly flowers, rose-
mary and lavender. Throw in some marjoram, savory and wild
thyme. Add the juice and peel of three lemons.
Boil together for four minutes. Strain and dry for fifteen days and
no longer. Sprinkle on the pillow of the marriage bed.

—After a medieval remedy for impotence

THEY SAT IN THE DOCTOR'S WAITING ROOM, HARDLY LOOKING AT ONE
another. She was intently reading a woman's magazine, he
puffed on his pipe. Finally their turn came to go in.

Gail and Jim R. wanted a baby. They had been married for
six years, and had stopped using any form of birth control three
years ago. So far nothing had happened. Could Dr. Don Sloan
help them with their problem?

Dr. Sloan started to outline the lengthy program of tests
necessary to determine why a particular couple may be infertile.
Then he began to ask a few general questions.

Was she regular? What surgical operations, if any?

Any venereal diseases?

The answers came fast and smoothly. She menstruated as
regularly as if she were a clock. No noteworthy illnesses. No
abdominal surgery. No history of TB or VD.

The questions continued.

How often did they have intercourse?

Once every two or three weeks, was the answer.

"Is that often enough for you?" Dr. Sloan asked.

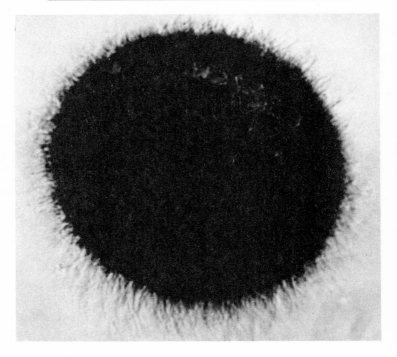

Ovum at the moment of fertilization ringed by sperm cells. Original magnified 1000 times. (Photo courtesy of Landrum B. Shettles, M.D., Randolph, Vermont)

Apparently it was, because Gail said she did not care that much for sex.

Though he did not tell them right away, Dr. Sloan felt that he had already hit the nail on the head. He also knew that it would take a lot of exploration to find out why this extremely attractive couple did not enjoy each other sexually.

Sexual dysfunction is much more frequent than might be suspected. According to Dr. Helen Kaplan Singer, a noted Manhattan sex therapist, about half of all couples have a sexual problem of one kind or another in the course of their relation-

ship and it is the major problem in 15 percent of couples suffering from "infertility." Yet it is often overlooked because both
the physician and the patients are very uncomfortable talking
about sex.

Most physicians unfortunately are still ill prepared to deal
with sexual problems. Until very recently the discussion of
sexual dysfunctions and their treatment was not part of a regular medical school curriculum, and in many places it still isn't.

At a recent course organized by the New York Fertility
Research Foundation and aimed at future infertility specialists,
Dr. Sloan cautioned his audience to be very good at listening to
their patients during the initial visit.

"It is going to take a doctor who is very comfortable in this
area to allow patients to feel reassured enough to talk about sex
in the office. If you communicate embarrassment, your patients
will get the message," he said. "They will not reveal important
things, or they may seek help elsewhere. You must convince the
patients right away that in sex there is no such thing as normal
and abnormal. If your patients convert their complaints into
organic symptoms, valuable time will be spent treating these
but missing what is behind them."

There are many cases of patients who for years submitted
to all kinds of time-consuming, expensive tests without anybody ever asking them how often they had intercourse.

Like all matters that involve a large psychological component, sexual dysfunction ranges from occasional to mild to severe to total. An added stressful situation such as pressure from
a job, or the need to have sex on schedule so as to produce a
child, are bound to exacerbate an existing dysfunction and even
create one that did not previously exist.

Much progress has been made in recent years in treating
these disorders. According to Dr. Sloan, who is the founding
president of the Eastern Association for Sex Therapy, the majority of patients can be helped by currently available methods
of sex therapy.

Female Problems

For decades after Queen Victoria ascended to the throne of Great Britain women were supposed to endure the sexual act with fortitude, thinking only of the pleasure they would eventually derive from motherhood. The influence of the good Queen was so strong that it took middle-class women fifty years to recover. Then it again slowly became permissible for a woman to admit that sex could be fun.

Better, safer methods of birth control, and Women's Lib came along, and today one can hardly pick up a woman's magazine without finding an article extolling the pleasures of multiple orgasm or detailing ways of enjoying oneself further in bed.

Yet some women are still very ignorant about the facts of life. Parents still have trouble talking frankly with their children, especially their daughters, about sex. Also, in this age of sexual enlightenment it is especially difficult for teenagers, let alone grown women, to admit their ignorance and ask questions

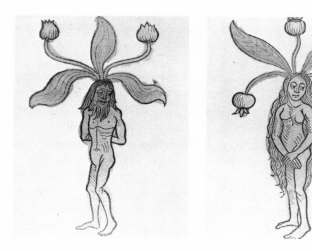

The mandrake plant, which was believed to come in a male and female form, was long thought to cure impotence and infertility as well as all the other ills of the lovelorn. It was a standard ingredient of aphrodisiacs. These German woodcuts were made in 1491. (Courtesy of National Library for Medicine, Bethesda, Maryland)

to which they feel they ought to know the answers.

In his practice Dr. Sloan is constantly surprised by how little some of his otherwise well-educated patients know about sexual matters. Sometimes, though rarely, ignorance of the sexual act is profound. Every gynecologist recalls seeing a few patients complaining of childlessness, whose hymen was intact —evidently the marriage was never even consummated.

The specific female disorders of sexuality that play a role in infertility are painful intercourse (dyspareunia), aversion to any type of sexual contact, and vaginismus. The last is characterized by such extreme constriction of the vaginal muscles as to prevent penetration of the penis or even the examining finger of the physician. But a patient often suffers from a combination of these three types of dysfunction.

A woman may also fail to respond to stimulus with adequate lubrication of her vagina. This has been described as the female equivalent of male impotence. However, just as most men can report an occasional such episode, women should not be upset if they occasionally fail to turn on to their partner.

Most women with a sexual dysfunction nevertheless manage to have intercourse. For some, however, the sex act is so distasteful that consciously or unconsciously the couple will copulate too infrequently to produce a child.

This was the case of Gail and Jim R. Gail came from a very sheltered home where sex was seldom talked about. From early on she absorbed the fact that women should be demure, polite, and passive, and that "nice" girls do not think of, talk about, or engage in sex.

Being so conditioned she shied away from sex talk with her friends, and turned a deaf ear to "street knowledge." All that did not prevent her from being a most attractive, flirtatious, and somewhat seductive young woman, who seemed to know much more about lovemaking than she really did.

Gail and Jim had a rather long courtship and engagement during which physical contact was kept at a minimum. Gail made it clear that she wanted to restrict herself until after marriage. Both believed that they would have an active sex life after they set up house, but the marriage license did little to overcome Gail's inhibition.

The R.'s never talked about their marital difficulties, and grew more and more distant from one another both physically and emotionally.

Instead of admitting that she might be partially responsible for their plight, Gail suggested that she had had more fun during a totally fictitious premarital affair. At parties she flirted wildly with a colleague of her husband. Jim not only felt deprived sexually, but also rejected. He retaliated by humiliating his wife in public. Their relationship became bitter, while the pressures for producing children grew stronger.

Friends and young relatives became parents, and their own parents wanted to graduate to grandparenthood. Reluctantly Gail and Jim had intercourse every two or three weeks, but the desired heir was not conceived. Now they wanted to know what to do.

After a few initial tests indicating that there was no obvious physical cause of infertility, Dr. Sloan recommended a course in marital sex therapy, which is mostly carried out by male and female co-therapists modifying the method developed by Dr. William H. Masters and Virginia E. Johnson of St. Louis. As compared to the more classical forms of psychotherapy the treatment is short—three to four weeks—with occasional follow-up visits over the next two years.

"We had to teach the R.'s that sex is a form of communication," Dr. Sloan explained. "In this particular case the young woman really needed a lot of basic education. She had never taken a good look at her genitalia, and she felt they were secret, painful parts of her body. We also taught them the importance of being honest with one another."

As an extreme example of how some couples conceal crucial information from one another, Dr. Sloan cites one patient who told him, when seen alone during an initial interview, that she was not the least surprised at their infertility since she had secretly been wearing an IUD for two years!

Male Problems

Throughout history it has been stressed that manliness and potency go hand in hand. Sometimes a man had to prove his virility publicly. It used to be customary, in some Arab lands, for the wedding guests to stay until the bridegroom showed the blood-stained sheet—proof of his manhood and his bride's chastity—from the window of the bridal chamber.

Even today a boy is expected to know much more about sex than a girl, and he is also expected to "perform" at a very early age. Yet deeply ingrained taboos against masturbation, the demands of peer groups, traumatic first sexual encounters, fear of failure, or homosexual leanings often put a man under enough pressure to result in impotence.

There are three major types of male sexual dysfunction: impotence and terminal impotence; premature ejaculation; and retarded ejaculation.

The word "impotence" comes from the Latin *impotentia*—meaning lack of power. Medically, impotence is defined as the inability of the male to achieve and/or maintain an erection sufficient for introducing his penis into the vagina. Terminal impotence refers to the loss of an erection after intromission but before ejaculation. Together the conditions affect about 10 to 15 percent of men who are infertile.

Premature ejaculation, which can be so severe that ejaculation occurs almost simultaneously with erection, is even more common than impotence.

Least common among the major sexual dysfunctions, but most frustrating, is retarded ejaculation, or the inability to complete an ejaculation in the vagina.

There is nothing very new about impotence and various other forms of sexual dysfunction.

In a recent article in *Penthouse Forum* magazine Dr. Sloan and Lillian Africano stated that:

Historically, men have experienced the problem throughout the centuries. The ancient Greeks pre-

scribed treatment for impotence, while Tolstoy
wrote about impotence in the Russian court. King
George III sought help for his problem from the famous physician John Hunter, and the legendary Don
Juan tried to cope with his problem by seducing
every woman he met. Even males of the supposedly
idyllic society of Polynesia experience impotence as
well as a form of performance anxiety.

Treatments for impotence are as old and varied
as the malady itself. Since the condition is seldom
discussed, and certainly is a man's best kept secret,
there are few statistics on the success rate of the
remedies.

It is generally felt by infertility specialists that
behavioral therapy, using a dual sex therapy team,
offers the best and quickest results for patients who
desire to overcome sexual dysfunction.

Dr. Sloan recalled one of the first couples suffering from infertility that he treated.

"It was almost a classic case.

"They had come all the way from Boston to see me. He
was a longshoreman who had worked his way up the hierarchy
of the union and by now he was quite a powerful boss. He
looked the part: tall, handsome, powerful, full of 'machismo.'

"Yet he was impotent, and since the couple was devoutly
Catholic, procreation was a vital part of their marriage.

"So he buried his pride, and shame, and came to see me.
He was very put down and it was difficult, at first, to deal with
the sexuality and impotence of a man who had that kind of
physique.

"But the couple did beautifully, much better indeed than
some of my more sophisticated patients.

"This early case really convinced me that sex therapy is
a very useful tool," Dr. Sloan concluded.

Sixty percent of all cases of impotence respond to behavioral therapy. The success rates for the treatment of premature

ejaculation is even higher (80 to 90 percent), whereas rates for retardate ejaculation are again 60 percent.

No matter what form of therapy the couple decides on, it is certain that treatment will begin with a verbal exploration of why the affected partner has trouble performing during intercourse.

"We often have trouble making a sexually dysfunctional infertile couple realize that there is much more to sex than simply making a baby," Dr. Sloan said. "Sex is a form of communication, a way of 'talking' to one another. When it breaks down, a couple starts to reject one another. They may choose to insult each other's families, to forget birthdays, to burn the dinner. Usually they end up by becoming openly hostile.

"I often start out by asking my patients whether 'buying' a baby would resolve their problem, or whether they are interested in repairing their relationship. I point out that many other factors are involved in conception and that they may not succeed in becoming parents even if they make love every day. Often it is only if they are willing to make a commitment to honesty with one another that we succeed in overcoming their sexual dysfunction."

A surprisingly large number of men suffering from retardate ejaculation are either unconsciously afraid of impregnating their wives or have taught themselves the practice of coitus interruptus (withdrawal) so well that they now seem unable to rid themselves of the habit.

To a large extent therapy is aimed at making people comfortable with their own likes and dislikes. Some couples are helped simply by changing their lovemaking patterns, by enabling them to become less anxious about the entire problem, and perhaps by introducing some erotica into their lives.

Most couples who specifically seek out the services of a sex therapist have already decided that they need more extensive professional help.

Apart from education about sexual matters and elucidation of why there is a problem, dual sex therapy concentrates on what are called "sensate-focus" exercises.

Patients are taught that past an initial threshold, nobody has voluntary control over their sexual responses. Beyond a certain point erection and ejaculation, relaxation of the vagina and lubrication, are as natural as breathing in and breathing out. One can, however, learn not to respond to certain stimuli and become sexually disabled. All behavioral techniques are aimed at unlearning destructive ways of doing things.

Though each sex therapy team uses their own specific method, adapted to the individual needs of the patient, the idea is to remove the couple from the stresses and strains of everyday life and have them concentrate on giving themselves and each other sensual pleasure.

The exercises are programmed from day to day. There is much emphasis on masturbation, and intercourse is postponed until the couple has learned, or relearned, to communicate on a verbal, emotional, and sexual level.

After the initial sexual barriers have been lowered, the sex therapy team will tackle the specific dysfunctional problems affecting each patient.

The preferred treatment for premature ejaculation, for instance, is to teach the woman to squeeze the shaft of the penis in such a manner as to delay the outpouring of the sperm. Gradually her partner will acquire new control.

Retarded ejaculation is one of the most difficult dysfunctions to treat. It often involves teaching the man to overcome the problem with self-stimulation (masturbation) exercises.

Recently Dr. Sloan treated a couple that had used withdrawal as a method of birth control for years. "The man delayed his ejaculation so successfully for so many years that when they wanted to have a baby he could no longer reverse the process.

"He was a most ambitious young man," Dr. Sloan recalled, "working during the day as a bank clerk, going to school at night, always attempting to better himself. The couple saw very little of one another. Often he came home so late that he slept on the couch so as not to disturb his wife.

"When the baby-problem became acute, he started to become very reproachful, accusing his wife of not being understanding enough of him and not cherishing him as a sexual partner. He felt that all she wanted of him now was a baby.

"During therapy we managed to teach this man, who was fortunate because he was able to ejaculate upon masturbation, gradually to associate ejaculation with his wife. I presume that unless they had another infertility problem, they are now happy parents."

Sometimes, though more rarely now than fifteen years ago, couples with sexual dysfunction will either refuse to take or will "flunk" a sex therapy course. In that case they might opt for having the woman inseminated with the husband's sperm obtained by masturbation (homologous artificial insemination). But the solution is far from ideal, since a satisfactory sex life is an integral part of every good marriage, which in turn is a necessary "soil" for growing happy children.

Like all those involved with infertility patients, Dr. Sloan derives a great deal of satisfaction from his practice. He recalls one couple he treated a number of years ago, who had unsuccessfully tried to have intercourse for a number of years in spite of much goodwill on the part of both. One day soon after they had completed his course, he received a long-distance call. "I'm calling you from a phone booth," the man said. "We just left the doctor's office and Marilyn's pregnancy test was positive. It will take us an hour to drive home," the future father went on, "and we just couldn't wait that long to let you know we made it."

16

ARTIFICIAL INSEMINATION

Maternity is a matter of fact—
Paternity is a matter of speculation.

—H. Gideon Wells

INTRODUCING SPERM CELLS INTO THE GENITAL TRACT OF THE FEMALE by means of a syringe or other mechanical means instead of through the genital organ of the male is called artificial insemination.

Artificial insemination is carried out most often with sperm obtained from an unrelated man. This is known as Artificial Insemination (with) Donor Sperm, or AID for short. In special cases the husband's sperm can be used. This is called Artificial Insemination (with) Homologous, or husband, sperm; AIH for short. The AID procedure is used when the husband is infertile and the wife is believed fertile; AIH is used when the husband's sperm is of poor quality.

Though the principle of artificial insemination has been known for centuries and the method has been used occasionally in man for about 100 years, the subject is still one of the most hushed up in medicine.

Some specialists compare the acceptance of artificial insemination today to that of contraception some fifty years ago.

As the late Dr. Sophie Kleegman, one of New York's leading infertility specialists, said in 1966: "Any change in custom or practice [related to sex, conception, and contraception] has always elicited a response from established custom and law of horrified negation at first; then negation without horror; then slow and gradual curiosity, study, evaluation, and finally a very slow, but steady acceptance."

Artificial insemination has been used in animal breeding for centuries. A tale of how a man got the prize stallion of his arch rival to ejaculate onto a piece of cloth, and subsequently used the semen to impregnate a mare, was recorded in 1322.

The first documented case of human insemination took place in England somewhere between 1776 and 1799. Ten more cases were reported in France in 1833. Dr. Marion Sims—who also developed the Sims-Huhner postcoital test that is still used today—was the first U.S. physician to write about artificial insemination in 1866.

In all these cases the wife was inseminated with the semen of her husband (AIH). Artificial insemination with donor sperm (AID) made its debut in America in the 1890s, when it was used in the greatest secrecy by Robert L. Dickinson, one of the most innovative gynecologists of his time.

It is really not surprising that artificial insemination is not readily discussed. Sexual prowess and fertility are almost synonymous with masculinity, and neither partner is likely to admit that the husband is not able to impregnate his wife.

This attitude is so deeply ingrained that most women are relieved to discover that *they* are the partner responsible for whatever infertility problem the couple may have. Fertility per se, be it male or female, is unrelated to a person's ability to be a good and passionate lover. The proof of this is that men and women who have undergone vasectomies or tubal ligations continue to have a very satisfactory sex life.

There are two other reasons for the reluctance to discuss artificial insemination.

As it is not customary or necessary to tell a test-tube baby of its provenance, it is best that as few people as possible are aware of the biological truth. This decreases the likelihood that the child will be told about it later in life.

CONSENT SLIP

Date: ————————————

We,———————————— being husband and wife and cohabiting as such, and being over twenty-one years old and residing at———————————— of our own free will and volition do request Dr.———————————— that he inseminate Mrs.———————————— , one of the undersigned herein, artificially with sperm of a male selected, or to be selected, by the same Dr.———————————— .

We make this request since we realize that Mr.———————————— is hopelessly sterile though not impotent, adequate laboratory tests having been performed, and further, because we are extremely anxious to have a child and we feel that our mental happiness and well being will be greatly enhanced by this artificial insemination. We understand that more than one attempt at artificial insemination may be required and there is no representation on the part of Dr.———————————— as to the number of attempts. We fully understand that Dr.———————————— does not or did not represent or warrant that a pregnancy or full term pregnancy will result from such artificial insemination, and further under no circumstances will we demand that the name of the donor of such such sperm be divulged.

We release the said Doctor of any and all responsibility in the event that the issue that may result from said artificial insemination is abnormal in any respect.

————————————————————
————————————————————

WITNESS: ————————————

Legal forms like this one are used by physicians performing artificial insimination.

The second reason for secrecy is that the legal status of donor-inseminated babies has not yet been clearly resolved. In 1964, Georgia was the first state to consider such children legitimate, provided the husband or the wife signed the appropriate papers. Some states followed suit, but the issue has not yet been resolved in all states of the Union.

Artificial Insemination Husband (Homologous)—AIH

Artificial insemination using the husband's sperm is useful when his sperm is of borderline quality, when the wife's cervical mucus is "hostile" and treatment to make it "friendly" has failed, when the husband is frequently away on business trips at about ovulation time, and when he is impotent or cannot ejaculate during regular coitus.

When the quality of the husband's sperm cells is poor or if his sperm count is low (from 8 million to 20 million per c.c.), his wife may be impregnated by collecting several specimens over a period of time. These specimens are stored by freezing and are kept ready for use at the appropriate time.

The first part of a man's ejaculate usually contains the greatest concentration of sperm. Use of one or more of these first portions (split ejaculate) for the insemination of the woman accounts for the success of AIH as compared with intercourse.

Before resorting to AIH, the quality (sperm density) of the sperm must be evaluated. Poor results are obtained if less than 50 percent of the sperm are motile or lack good forward progression. A large proportion of abnormal sperm is also suspect.

A pregnancy rate of 22 percent has been achieved with low-count, good-quality sperm. In all cases the man must provide a specimen once or twice a week, which is then examined under the microscope and stored in a sperm bank until ready for use.

The specimen must be as fresh as possible, and it is often advisable that it be ejaculated in the laboratory where the freezing will take place.

The sperm is then concentrated by careful spinning in a cold centrifuge—the heavy sperm will settle at the bottom. Before they are frozen, the sperm are mixed with substances that will protect them during storage. Such *cryo* (cold) protective agents include egg yolk and glycerine.

The specimens are frozen in a plastic straw and stored in a sperm bank—a big metal container filled with liquid nitrogen, at a temperature of −197°C. When needed, several specimens are thawed and pooled.

Physicians attribute some of the good results obtained with this method to the fact that many patients with low-count sperm do occasionally produce a good specimen. Normally there is a small chance that such a specimen will be produced just precisely when the wife is fertile.

Such infrequent high-quality specimens may account for the fact that some couples, infertile for years on end, suddenly manage to achieve parenthood unaided. Today modern medicine simply lends nature a helping hand. Artificial insemination with the husband's sperm is also useful when the cervix of the wife prevents normal progression of the sperm. Such a defect shows up in the postcoital test.

If treatment with drugs fails to correct this condition, the cervical mucus can be bypassed.

Sexual maladjustment, including the inability of the husband to ejaculate in his wife, occurs more frequently than is generally known. Artificial insemination can be used to resolve

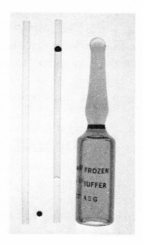 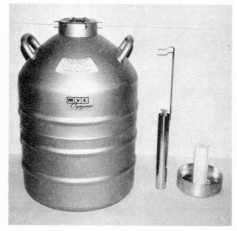

Sperm cells are stored in small straws at about − 196° C. in a container filled with liquid nitrogen.

the biological, if not the psychological problems, of such couples.

One of the most successful cases ever treated at the New York Fertility Research Institute involved a patient who had come from a distance reporting that her husband was unable to have an intravaginal ejaculation. After listening to some explanations of the facts of life, she returned home. A few months later she wrote a letter informing her doctor that she had inseminated herself with a turkey baster and now was pregnant!

Artificial Insemination with Donor Sperm (AID)

The demand for artificial insemination with donor sperm has increased phenomenally since the early 1970s. Dr. Wayne Decker now performs about 200 inseminations a month, as compared to a mere 2 to 3 in 1970.

Better birth control methods, liberal abortion laws, and the fact that unwed mothers often opt for keeping their babies has made the method more attractive to couples who might otherwise have decided to adopt. Yet according to Dr. Wayne Decker, AID is rarely the first choice of patients who seek his help for this purpose.

Though figures are hard to come by, it is estimated that 10,000 to 20,000 babies are fathered each year by AID in the United States. Considering that men are responsible for 30 to 40 percent of all infertile marriages, this birth figure is low; it can be expected to increase further as patients become more used to the idea.

Increased acceptability also rests on the fact that husband and wife seem to be increasingly capable of separating the pleasures of intimacy associated with sexual love from the mechanics of AID. Many couples feel that though it may be regretful that their offspring will not have both their genes, half a loaf is much better than none. Also, and perhaps most important, a woman who carries her own AID baby can experience all the joys and hardships of pregnancy and birth.

There are nevertheless all kinds of psychological, legal,

and religious questions associated with artificial insemination.

All physicians who practice AID will insist that both the husband and wife come to an initial lengthy interview. This gives the physician a chance to evaluate the strength of the couple's marriage, and gives the prospective parents a chance to talk about their hopes and fears.

Dr. Wayne Decker observed that by the time a couple appears in the office seeking information about artificial insemination, they are emotionally and psychologically ready to accept donor insemination. According to him they have usually weighed the pros and cons of the procedure, and look forward to its successful outcome.

If the physician feels that either partner has some reservations, it is advisable to schedule another appointment a month or so later, so that the subject can again be explored.

Some physicians also find that a rap session during which the patients express their views is very helpful. Dr. Wayne Decker has arranged group therapy sessions for some of his patients.

As society develops more diversified roles, and lifestyles for both men and women change, artificial insemination is also requested by single women and female homosexual couples. The decision as to whether to accede to such requests is up to the physician.

Dr. Wayne Decker feels that single women who wish to become mothers are suitable candidates, provided that they are fully aware of the long-term problems and pleasures of parenthood and can provide for a child economically.

Before such inseminations are carried out, the physician should investigate the lifestyle of the prospective mother. It is important that single women have an accepting, extended family and a secure social position. Under such circumstances there is no reason to assume that the offspring will fare worse than if the mother were divorced, widowed, or had opted for bringing up her out-of-wedlock child.

Artificial insemination also involves some legal problems. Documents must be signed by both the husband and the wife.

These essentially state that the patients understand the procedure and problems involved, that the woman requests the procedure, that she will accept the responsibility for any abnormal or defective child, and that the couple will accept the offspring as their own.

The couple may also wish to discuss their decision with their religious counselor. The Protestant Church has not taken a firm stand on artificial insemination one way or another, whereas the orthodox Jewish, Lutheran, most Anglican sects, and the Catholic religions are all strongly opposed to it. If one is to judge, however, by parishioners' nonadherence to their church's dictates on birth control, the use of artificial insemination will increase regardless.

Donor Selection

Donors should always be selected by the physician from a healthy pretested group of men known to be fertile. Too many potential problems exist when the donor is selected by or known to the woman or her mate. An attempt is always made to select donors who resemble the husband from a physical point of view. At one point an effort was made at selecting particularly gifted donors. Doctors who pioneered AID in America insisted that their test-tube babies be brought in about once a year to undergo various intelligence tests.

Other early variants included the pooling of sperm obtained from several donors, and even adding some of the husband's sperm. In this way nobody knew who the biological father really was. Furthermore there was always the outside chance that the ovum was fertilized by the man the baby would call Daddy.

Today most of these practices have been abandoned, and physicians content themselves with matching the donor to the physical characteristics of the father of fact as far as height, skin, hair, and eye color are concerned. This has been greatly facilitated by the advent of sperm banks where frozen sperm can be kept for months and years on end.

Donors are now paid for their services. They are carefully selected. Most are married and have normal children. Medical students, interns, and residents are often used because they are more aware of their family's medical history and of the importance of providing accurate data. In order to avoid accidental incest among the children they have fathered, the use of their sperm is restricted. They are not told whether their sperm took, and since a woman usually requires more than one insemination a certain element of mystery remains.

Using donor sperm whose identity is known to the physician has the additional advantage that parents who come back for another baby can ask for the same biological father.

Technique

The actual technique of insemination is simple and entirely painless. The pattern follows that of normal intercourse as much as possible.

The time of ovulation is pinpointed as carefully as possible by means of the BBT chart, by vaginal smears carried out around ovulation time, or by the behavior *(spinnbarkeit)* of the cervical mucus. Most women undergoing artificial insemination are somewhat anxious, and even those who usually ovulate as regularly as clockwork become somewhat erratic. Spontaneous regular ovulation usually resumes within one to three cycles. Some physicians also ensure regular ovulation by treating all their patients with clomiphene citrate.

Once the crucial time has been ascertained, the patient is inseminated three to four times on consecutive days.

A straw-sized metal cannula is attached to a glass syringe. The semen specimen is drawn into the syringe and deposited in the vagina. Most physicians prefer to stream semen over the cervical os. Semen that collects in the vagina is reaspirated and run over the os three or four more times.

After the insemination the patient is asked to remain on the table for about twenty minutes. Sometimes a special foam rubber plastic-covered cylinder is inserted in the vagina to hold the seminal fluid. This tampon is to be removed by the patient after approximately three hours.

Patients are also advised to have intercourse shortly after insemination, not so much to add doubt about who the real father is as to strengthen the husband's sense of participation in the creative process.

Outcome

Good results are obtained with both frozen and fresh semen. Approximately 25 percent of the patients will be pregnant after the first cycle, 50 percent after six months, and 80 percent within one year. Few pregnancies occur after one year. Put in other terms, there will be one pregnancy for every twelve to fourteen inseminations. These rates of conception are very similar to those observed in the normal population.

The outcome of the pregnancies initiated with artificial insemination are very similar to those resulting from normal intercourse. If anything there are somewhat fewer abnormalities or malformations, probably because inseminations are always done with highly fertile sperm at the optimum time, before the ovum has had a chance to age.

Once pregnancy is achieved, the couple usually selects another physician to deliver the baby. In the first place most artificial insemination specialists practice in large urban centers. Many also have a restricted practice. Finally, and most important, a physician who is unaware of the biological parentage of the infant can sign the birth certificate that lists the husband of the mother as the biological father without knowingly falsifying the data.

The AID Family (Psychological Consequences)

Because it is such a well-kept secret, little is known about families who owe their existence to AID.

The late Dr. Alan Guttmacher surveyed 300 such families and found that they were in better than average shape as far as their mental health was concerned. At least none of the couples he investigated had been divorced.

In the cases that are known, both parents accepted the child as their own. One mother reported that both she and her husband had forgotten the child's origin to such an extent that they always kept wondering from whom their son had acquired such-and-such a trait. And this is not surprising. After all, the physical genes are only responsible in small part for what any human being will turn out to be. Love, acceptance, the example of all those who take part in the rearing of the child will in the end be the determining factors.

One of the few test-tube babies who was told of her biological provenance when she was nineteen wrote that the knowledge had never made any difference. She was grateful for the trouble her parents had taken to give her life, and she had quite naturally absorbed the rich cultural roots of her immigrant family. In fact she felt that her parents' decision to solve their problem in a then unusual way was a positive, somewhat liberating experience for her entire family.

17

SPERM KILLERS— IMMUNE FACTORS AS A CAUSE OF INFERTILITY

Curiouser and Curiouser!

—Lewis Carroll

THE WAR BETWEEN THE SEXES GOES BACK TO ADAM AND EVE. BUT UNTIL recent times nobody had realized that some women actually develop a factor that can destroy or inactivate sperm cells, and that some men are "allergic" to their own semen.

It sometimes seems as if there are mythological precedents to most infertility problems. An old legend has it that the semen of King Minos of Crete contained snakes and scorpions that not only were injurious to his sexual partners, but kept him from siring normal children.

He thus refrained from consummating his marriage to Parsiphae, the beautiful daughter of the King of the Sun.

Minos is said to have circumvented the difficulty by shedding his first ejaculate into a condom made from the bladder of a goat. This apparently purified his seed, because he then successfully fathered four sons and four daughters.

Millennia have passed since Minos' time, but today condoms are sometimes used as a means of treatment for this particular cause of infertility.

The body of a woman "unfriendly" to her own husband's

sperm is not more kindly disposed to anyone else's. The phenomenon is not a matter of psychology, but related to the immune system that plays such an important role in health and disease.

In order to survive in a hostile world, nature has equipped us with a mechanism with which we can make short shrift of most infectious agents and reject outright anything as totally foreign as somebody else's heart or kidney.

We wage this defensive war by means of thousands of antibodies that we seem to be able to tailor-make upon demand whenever a special need arises. These antibodies then combine with the "invader" (called an antigen), which can be a virus, a foreign protein or, as we shall see, a sperm cell.

We are so ready to manufacture these antibodies that it is perhaps astonishing that women, and other mammals, are actually able to carry their offspring through weeks and months of pregnancy. Since a fetus is very much like a foreign graft, pregnancy is one of the mysteries of immunology.

The immune system, however, is far from perfect. It misfires often, and many major and minor diseases—from hay fever to multiple sclerosis, rheumatoid arthritis, and perhaps even cancer—are at least partially caused by a malfunction of the immune system.

Infertility seems to be no exception. Several studies of large numbers of couples with an unexplained infertility problem have shown that about 17 percent of the women have antibodies to sperm, as compared to 3 percent of pregnant or postpartum controls. Ten percent of men also have antibodies to sperm.

One of the groups who study the role that immunity plays in infertility is headed by Dr. Sidney Shulman at New York Medical College in New York. Dr. Shulman recommends that sperm antibody tests be done on patients with any long-term unexplained infertility, and especially on those who have repeated abnormal postcoital tests or a positive mucus-hostility test.

Antibodies are usually found in the serum part of the

blood. In our particular case they are found in the serum of the woman, or the man, and they also may be present in the cervical mucus or the seminal fluid surrounding the sperm cells. Each partner is tested for sperm antibodies. It is extremely rare for both members of a couple to have the same rather uncommon physiologically abnormal reaction, although this does occur.

Several tests are available to ascertain the presence of antibodies, and it is recommended that more than one method be used.

In one of the procedures a small diluted amount of the sample to be tested (serum, cervical mucus extract, or seminal plasma) is mixed with fresh, diluted semen (which can be the husband's or somebody else's). After several hours of incubation the specimen is examined under a microscope. Sperm antibodies will clump or agglutinate a portion of the sperm cells. The extent of the clumping is an indication of the amount of antibody present.

Sometimes the results of this test show a complete loss of motility of the sperm cells. This immobilization can also indicate the presence of sperm antibodies.

Antibodies are not always found in both serum and the other specimen examined. A number of women only have sperm antibodies in their cervical mucus and not in their serum, or vice versa.

There is as yet no explanation why some patients spontaneously develop antibodies to sperm. In experimental animals such antibodies do develop generally when sperm cell preparations are injected. Such "immunization" is one of the very promising new experimental methods of birth control now under investigation by Dr. Shulman and other scientists.

One hypothesis accounting for the spontaneous sperm antibodies found in women is based on the belief that some material derived from spermatozoa leaks through the walls of the vagina into the bloodstream, where it would act as if it had been injected on purpose.

This line of reasoning does not apply to men. However, Dr. Shulman and others speculate that in men the sperm antibodies may result from childhood infections, from mumps orchitis, or more probably from a partial or transitory obstruction of the vas deferens. It has been observed that 60 percent of men who have undergone vasectomy operations have sperm antibodies.

Treatment

Few methods of therapy are as yet available to patients whose infertility *may* be caused by sperm antibodies. Since the concentration of these decreases when the stimulant is removed, couples in whom the *woman* has the antibodies are instructed to use a condom whenever having intercourse in order to prevent sperm contact in the woman. Often the antibody concentration (titer) slowly drops to an acceptable level. Dr. Shulman recommends that the serum of such female partners should then be tested for sperm antibody every three months.

When the titer is as low as it will go, the fertile period of the woman is determined, and the couple is advised to have intercourse without using the condoms at the appropriate times. Though figures are hard to come by, it is said that 50 percent of the couples treated by this method conceived and had children.

The treatment of men is much more difficult, since they continue to be exposed to their own sperm.

Attempts are being made to remove sperm antibodies from the ejaculate, by washing the sperm cells and inseminating the female partner with the cleansed material. Insemination with split ejaculates—using only the first half of the semen, which is both richer in sperm and poorer in antibodies—has also been tested. Unfortunately neither method is often successful.

Another approach is to try to depress the entire spectrum of antibodies manufactured by the male partner by using corticosteroids. Until recently the method failed completely, but Dr. Shulman reports one spectacular success obtained in a couple with a long-standing infertility problem apparently caused by sperm antibodies present in the man.

This male patient was treated with large doses of the corticosteroid methylprednisolone during the early part of the female cycle. Appropriate tests revealed that the blood level of the husband's antibodies dropped considerably after treatment. After two months of such treatment the couple conceived, and though Dr. Shulman is "heady with excitement," he is the first to concede that more data are required before the method is acclaimed widely.

In summary, investigation of what role immunity plays in infertility is a new field. Much remains to be learned. It is at present believed that sperm antibodies play a role in 30 percent of patients with unexplained infertility, and other types of abnormal immune reaction probably also play a role. In view of the many causes of infertility already reviewed here this is only a relatively small number of people. But a better understanding of the role of immunity will be one more step in solving the dual problem of infertility and overfertility in the world.

18

WILL OUR BABY
BE NORMAL?

EVERYTHING SEEMED TO BE GOING SWIMMINGLY FOR HOWARD AND LILA Jones. He had just been promoted to account executive at his advertising agency; she loved being a kindergarten teacher. Her parents loved him; his parents loved her; they seemed to like everybody.

They had just moved from their small studio apartment to a two-family house in the suburbs because their first child was to be born in July, when Lila was through teaching for the year.

Everything was ready—a crib, a baby carriage, a small bathinette. Both "expectant" grandmothers had been knitting and Baby Jones would be a fashion plate.

But the baby never used any of these things. After she was born, it was discovered that she was profoundly retarded. The Joneses never took her home.

Much later, when Lila was at last able to talk about their misfortune, she said that she never once considered that "such a thing could happen to her."

Mental retardation and other birth defects are a major health problem which, like infertility, have only recently become "respectable." Acceptance is partially due to the fact that many famous people—the Kennedys, the Humphreys, Beverly Sills—have talked about the fact that they are the mothers, fathers, or grandparents of retarded or mentally disturbed children.

Birth defects have many causes. The cases that will concern us here are knitted into the genetic fabric of the fetus.

From a biochemical and genetic point of view living creatures are totally programmed. All the information pertaining to skin and eye color, hair, and blood type, right down to the last protein needed to keep the complex body chemistry going, is coded into long chemical molecules, called deoxyribonucleic acid, or DNA for short.

In man this DNA has been arranged into forty-six chromosomes, found in each cell of the body. Each chromosome is further subdivided into thousands of genes that mastermind and supervise particular human traits.

The science of genetics is very young. The chromosomes were discovered almost exactly 100 years ago, and can now easily be seen under a microscope. It was also shown over the next decades that the chromosomes consisted of DNA.

Nobody as yet has been able to see an individual gene, which is a small region on a particular chromosome; but scientists at present are busy mapping the chromosomes, discovering for instance that eye color is determined by such-and-such a region on such-and-such a chromosome.

In 1953 Drs. Francis H. C. Crick and James D. Watson showed that the DNA of the chromosomes was arranged as a set of double helixes that pulled apart (separated) during reproduction, each chain of DNA being able to direct the cell to make an exact copy of itself. This is how information is handed from cell to cell and from generation to generation. Most cells in the human body contain forty-six chromosomes. These are arranged into twenty-three pairs. During cell division, or *mitosis,* each chromosome in each pair copies itself exactly, and the two daughter cells again have twenty-three pairs of chromosomes.

There is one major exception to this general state of affairs

—the process of reproduction. Like all other cells of the body, the precursor cells of the ovum (oocyte) and of the sperm (spermatocyte) contain forty-six chromosomes arranged in twenty-three pairs. Before they mature into ova and spermatozoa, these cells undergo reduction division, or *meiosis,* a process by which the daughter cells retain only one of the two chromosomes of each pair. The mature ova and the spermatozoa each have only twenty-three single chromosomes.

During fertilization the twenty-three single chromosomes contributed by the mother merge with the twenty-three single chromosomes contributed by the father, resulting in a complete cell containing twenty-three pairs of chromosomes. This single cell—the fertilized ovum—will immediately divide, forming two, four, eight, sixteen cells. Within nine months a complete new human being will be born.

As in all complicated processes mistakes occur occasionally. During the fertilization of the egg by the sperm a defective seed, which will never grow into a healthy human being, is occasionally produced.

Fortunately for mankind most defects are so serious that the embryo is incapable of surviving, even within the sheltered atmosphere of the womb, for more than a couple of weeks. Ninety-eight percent of all defective conceptions are lost by abortion; only 2 percent are "healthy" enough to survive. Yet even this small percentage, according to the National Foundation March of Dimes, accounts for 200,000 defective babies born in America annually.

It is a rare couple that does not fear they may be the parents of such a child.

The scientists of human genetics have already learned enough to be able sometimes to predict before birth whether or not an unborn child is afflicted by certain genetic defects, thus offering the couple the possibility of an abortion. In order to understand how such defects can be diagnosed before birth, we have to learn a little more about genetics.

We have already pointed out that each cell contains twenty-three pairs of chromosomes. One of these twenty-three pairs is special. It is the sex chromosome pair. The X chromosome is the female chromosome, the Y the male chromosome. The X chromosome is larger than the Y chromosome.

The cells of a healthy woman always have two paired chromosomes (XX), the cells of a healthy man always have a paired X and Y chromosome (XY).

During meiosis the sex-chromosome pair, along with the other twenty-two chromosome pairs, undergoes reduction division. In men this will result in sperm cells, half of which will have X chromosomes and the other half Y chromosomes. Eventually these will mature into gynosperm (sperm carrying an X chromosome) and androsperm (sperm carrying a Y chromosome).

The oocyte of the woman, which has two X chromosomes to begin with, will also undergo reduction division. All mature ova, however, will carry one X chromosome, since women do not have Y chromosomes.

During fertilization there will be a merger of the X-chromosome-bearing ovum with either a Y-bearing androsperm or an X-bearing gynosperm. This results in cells with a full complement of forty-six chromosomes, approximately 50 percent of which are XY and 50 percent XX, thus maintaining an equal distribution of the sexes.

Geneticists have become very familiar with what human chromosomes look like under the microscope. The chromosomes of a cell can best be seen when the cell is dividing, because it is only then that they arrange themselves in an orderly fashion. Before they "sit" for their photographic portrait, they are stained with special dyes.

A technician cuts the photograph into pieces and arranges the individual pairs into a karyotype (*karyo* means nucleus, and indeed the chromosomes are contained in the nucleus of a cell).

In a karyotype the chromosome pairs are arranged according to size—the largest chromosome pair being number 1. The pairs are numbered from 1 to 22. The sex chromosome pair has no number.

Pairs 1 to 22 are called the *autosomal chromosomes*, or autosomes. Pair 23 is the sex chromosome pair.

If you ever have to become more deeply involved with genetics, you may hear such terms as autosomal recessive, autosomal dominant, and sex-linked. All this refers to the type of chromosome in which a particular "trait" is located, and whether it will be strong or weak.

Such terms do not necessarily relate to disease. Blue eyes, for instance, are autosomal recessive, meaning that the gene or genes for eye color are on a regular (autosomal) chromosome, rather than on a sex chromosome, and that blue eyes will only "show" (express themselves is the scientific term) provided each parent contributes a gene for blue eye color.

To you the various chromosomes may look alike. But scientists who are accustomed to looking at karyotypes are very quick to number the pairs and identify those that look abnormal. This has become even easier since the chromosomes are treated with special dyes that make them appear "banded."

As mentioned earlier, an error sometimes occurs during cell division. The chromosome pairs may not divide properly (nondysjunction) and the fertilized ovum may for instance contain an extra X chromosome (XXY).

In the most frequently noted genetic abnormality—mongolism or Down's Syndrome—chromosome "pair" number 21 contains *three* instead of *two* chromosomes. For this reason this birth defect is also called "trisomy 21."

Among the other genetic defects that have so far been identified the most well known is probably Turner's Syndrome. In this case the offspring has an abnormal sex chromosome pair. It may lack a second X or a Y chromosome and the sex chromosome pair reads OX. Women suffering from this very rare defect are short and have an abnormal sexual development.

Much attention recently has been paid to the also rare Klinefelter Syndrome, in which a male has one or more extra X chromosomes. These men are usually sterile, and may exhibit female characteristics such as enlarged breasts.

Most genetic defects that have been characterized scientifically so far are much more subtle than the two described

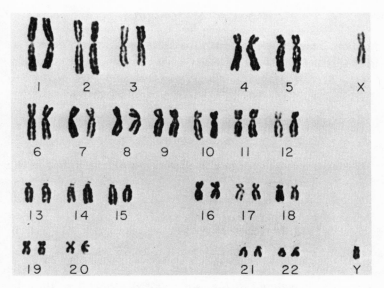

This is a normal karyotype. (Courtesy of March of Dimes)

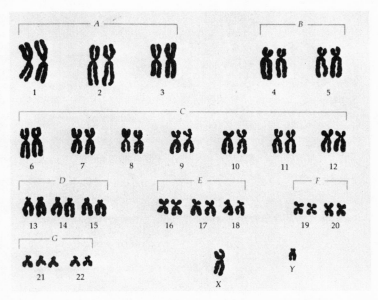

This is a karyotype of a person suffering from Down's Syndrome or trisomy 21.
(Courtesy of March of Dimes)

above. Geneticists today can diagnose such inborn defects as Tay-Sachs Disease, hemophilia, phenylketonuria, spina bifida, cystic fibrosis, and especially a rather common incompatibility between mother and child known as the Rh-factor.

Amniocentesis

Discovering that some genetic diseases can be identified in the karyotype was only half the battle. The other half was obtaining cells from the embryo, which was easier said than done. After all, before birth the fetus is well hidden inside the mother.

About forty years ago it was discovered that one could remove a small amount of amniotic fluid, in which the fetus is suspended. (The fluid and the fetus are enclosed in the amniotic sac—bag of waters.) In the late 1960s it was shown that the

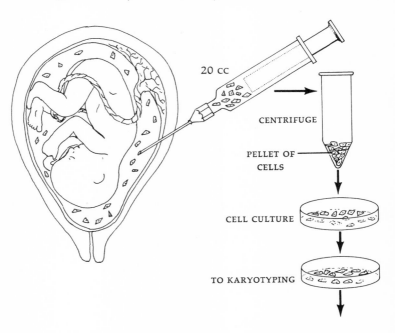

During amniocentesis a small amount of fluid is removed from the amniotic sac and analyzed.

amniotic fluid contains a few cells shed by the fetus.

Dr. Ernest Lieber, of the Division of Human Genetics, Long Island Jewish Hospital, Department of Pediatrics, in Great Neck, New York, tells his patients that these stray cells are very much like the ring found around the bathtub after one has taken a bath. The latter consists in part of cells shed from the skin of the bather. The fetus also discards some cells. Amniotic fluid can be removed without harming mother or child.

Each one of the cells obtained by amniocentesis contains a complete sample of the chromosomes of the fetus. When looked at under the microscope, they will reveal any abnormal chromosomal configuration. It is, however, impossible to look directly at the cells obtained during amniocentesis. Before they can be interpreted, the cells must be made to grow and divide in a suitable culture medium, because it is only during cell division that the chromosomes arrange themselves neatly in pairs.

When carried out at a reputable, well-equipped medical center, amniocentesis is a safe procedure. It is usually done between the fourteenth and sixteenth week of pregnancy. Most experts feel that it is best to first locate the exact position of the fetus and especially of the placenta, which supports the fetus during the nine months of pregnancy, by an ultrasonic scan.

After the scan the physician removes about 20 milliliters of amniotic fluid with a syringe via needle puncture through the abdominal wall. Some physicians give their patients a local anesthetic before removing the fluid; others do not because they believe that the needle used to inject the anesthetic hurts as much as that used to extract the fluid.

The major portion of the fluid removed from the amniotic sac is gently centrifuged so as to collect the cells in the bottom of the tube. The cells form a little pellet which is broken up and distributed into three to four plastic flasks. Serum and other essential nutrients are added. The cells start growing, but it takes about three weeks until there are enough of them so that they can be harvested, stained, photographed, and arranged in a karyotype.

One of the by-products of amniocentesis is that the parents learn the sex of their child. (Each cell of the body contains either an XX or an XY chromosome pair.)

Though gross chromosomal abnormalities can now often be detected during amniocentesis, some progress is being made in identifying other defects that may be reflected in the amniotic fluid itself. Several serious birth defects are caused by the presence or absence of a key chemical substance, or of one of the enzymes necessary to convert one key chemical substance into another. Today some of these diseases can be identified from careful analysis of the amniotic fluid.

Most parents can relax when they hear the results of the amniocentesis. In a study organized by the National Institutes of Health, out of 1,040 amniocenteses done at 9 medical centers between 1971 and 1973, on a high-risk group of women, only 45 fetuses showed any kind of abnormality. These included nineteen chromosomal abnormalities, fifteen metabolic abnormalities, and eleven males at risk of developing X-linked disease.

Amniocentesis is not infallible. In the above NIH study, there were five errors in predicting the sex of the child. Two children believed to be normal were born with Down's Syndrome, and one fetus believed to suffer from galactosemia—a serious but treatable metabolic disease—who was not aborted turned out to be normal.

Several birth defects, including sickle cell anemia and thalassemia—both affecting the blood—cannot easily be detected by amniocentesis. These defects must be identified in blood, and fetal blood is still very difficult to obtain without risking injury to the baby.

Medical genetics and genetic counseling do not only involve laboratory tests. Much information is derived from the pedigree or family tree of the parents and their relatives.

A case in point is Huntington's chorea, one of the most cruel diseases known to man. The illness manifests itself only after age thirty-five, when the future patient may already have parented children of his or her own. The disease, which affected folksinger Woody Guthrie, causes mental deterioration, irritability, premature senility, and uncontrollable body and muscle spasms.

The disease is inherited in an as yet unidentified autosomal dominant pattern. This means that all persons who carry the gene for the disease will have the disease. Since each child has half a chance of getting this particular chromosome from the affected parent, half the children of such a union will be afflicted.

Several important genetic defects are linked to the sex chromosomes. They are referred to as sex-linked diseases. In this case the disease will appear in one sex or the other.

Hemophilia—characterized by a clotting defect in the blood—is the prime example of a sex-linked genetic disease. The gene for hemophilia is located on an X chromosome. It only becomes expressed when the single defective X chromosome is *not neutralized* by a healthy X chromosome. This is why overt disease only occurs in males.

Matters are different in women. As a rule they do not have overt disease. (Hemophilia, in women, would result from two defective X chromosomes—one from the mother, one from the father—which is a rare occurrence indeed.) Half of the daughters of a woman with a defective X chromosome are carriers of the disease, and hand the disease on to future generations.

As it is still impossible to detect hemophilia by amniocentesis, a decision as to whether a pregnancy should be interrupted is mostly based on a thorough study of the family history. In this particular case parents may decide to abort a male fetus, who has a 50 percent chance of having overt disease, and preserve a female pregnancy, since the daughter, at worst, will be a carrier.

Barr Bodies

Geneticists have recently come up with another piece of scientifically important information—the Barr body, named after its discoverer Dr. M. L. Barr. In 1969 when he studied the nerve cells of cats, Dr. Barr noted that all the cells obtained from female cats had a speck of dark material in their nucleus, while the nuclei of the cells obtained from male cats did not have such specks.

Further investigation indicated that in mammals, including women, the nuclei of female cells have such Barr bodies. It turned out that this Barr body is the inactive stage of the second X chromosome each woman has.

If this extra chromosome were expressed biochemically, the woman would have a double dose of some of the enzymes and proteins whose manufacture is supervised by the X chromosome. Since men only have one X chromosome, they do not have any Barr bodies.

The presence of Barr bodies has become an important tool in the diagnosis of diseases characterized by extra numbers of X chromosomes like the Klinefelter Syndrome (men suffering from this condition *do* have Barr bodies). The absence of Barr bodies in a woman signifies that this patient lacks an X chromosome (Turner's Syndrome).

Barr bodies can be identified in every body cell. In practice the cells are usually obtained by gently scraping the cheek inside the mouth. They are then spread on a glass slide, stained, and examined under the microscope.

Sometimes testing for Barr bodies is done at birth when there is a question about the sexual identity of the child.

Sex Determination

There has been much discussion in popular literature as to the advantages for parents of choosing the sex of their child.

Amniocentesis, followed by abortion if the child turns out to be the "wrong" sex, presents such a possibility. This is, however, not the purpose of a procedure whose availability can save many people much grief. Most parents who for medical reasons, or age factors, submit to the procedure are overjoyed to be told that they will have a healthy baby, regardless of its sex.

Other means of planning the sex of the desired offspring

are being investigated. One promising method is based on the fact that sperm bearing an X chromosome, the gynosperm, is slightly heavier and rounder than the Y-chromosome-bearing sperm (androsperm). When sperm cells are diluted with special fluid and spun in a centrifuge, it might in the future be possible to separate these two types of sperm and use the desired gender for artificial insemination.

Dr. Landrum Shettles, who for a number of years worked at both Columbia University and at the New York Fertility Research Foundation, has attempted to perfect a method based on the time of intercourse by means of which parents could increase their chances of having either a male or a female child.

The reasoning behind the method is that the androsperm is lighter and more streamlined. It thus swims faster than the rounder, heavier gynosperm. The androsperm is also more sensitive to acid and has a somewhat shorter lifespan.

If intercourse is scheduled so that it takes place at or shortly after ovulation time, the chances of having a male offspring are enhanced since the fast-swimming androsperm will get to the egg earlier than the gynosperm. On the other hand the gynosperm seem to be longer lived because they are more resistant to the acid environment of the vagina. Scheduling intercourse a few days before ovulation time may thus increase the chances of producing a female child.

Though sex determination may present certain advantages from the angle of population control, since people would presumably stop trying to have children until they attained the correct mix, psychologists, physicians, and other concerned persons object on ethical grounds.

One reason is that because of a cultural bias most parents would choose to start their families with a boy. It has recently been shown that first-born children have more than their share of very specific character traits, including a gift for leadership, high achievement, creativity, and self-reliance. If the population figures were altered so as to reduce the number of first-born girls, there would be fewer women with these very desirable qualities.

19

PARENTHOOD
AFTER
THIRTY-FIVE

And the Lord visited Sarah as He had said, and the Lord did unto Sarah as He had spoken.

For Sarah conceived, and bore Abraham a son in his old age, at the set time of which God had spoken to him . . .

And Abraham was a hundred years old, when his son Isaac was born unto him. And Sarah said: "God hath made laughter for me; every one that heareth will laugh on account of me," and she said: "Who would have said unto Abraham that Sarah should give children suck? For I have borne him a son in his old age."

—Genesis 21

IN 1923, WHEN SHE WAS FORTY-TWO YEARS OLD, MRS. THERESE LOEBL felt rather ill. Her stomach just would not settle down. Since she believed that she had overindulged during the Christmas holidays, she delayed going to the doctor. When she finally went, she was dumbfounded when told that she might be pregnant. Her surprise was understandable. She had been married at the age of nineteen and had never used any form of birth control.

In due time Mrs. Loebl delivered a healthy boy by Caesarean section, which then was a major operation. At his birth her doctors discovered that she had a bicornate uterus, which might have been responsible for her low fertility.

Had she been infertile today, Mrs. Loebl would probably have explored the reason for her condition much earlier. She also would have worried whether her child would be normal.

We know today that older mothers do have a higher incidence of abnormal children, and gynecologists are quick to point out that a woman should if possible start her family before she is thirty.

But one is not always able to plan one's life to perfection. Health problems, including those associated with infertility, marital status, career decisions, and unplanned pregnancies, all make it sometimes necessary or desirable to have a child later in life. We shall thus explore what is known about pregnancy and childbirth toward the end of the fertile years and attempt to separate fact from fiction.

All scientists agree that it is biologically best for a woman to bear her children between the ages of twenty and thirty-four. The risk to both mother and child increases on either side of this age bracket. However, other factors, such as good medical care, can balance these disadvantages. Thus having a child beyond the optimum age is more dangerous in an underdeveloped country than in one with a relatively high standard of living.

There are several types of problems connected with having children after the age of thirty-five: decreased fertility; increased risk during pregnancy and delivery; increased risk to the fetus and child; and various psychological factors.

Before we consider these subjects in detail, let us begin by stating that in absolute terms there is no great risk in being an "older" mother. In other words the overwhelming majority of expectant mothers over thirty-five have normal pregnancies and deliver normal babies, which they take great pleasure in watching grow to adulthood.

In a way people are much younger today than they used to be. In the United States and in western Europe life expectancy at birth has risen from forty-one years in 1840 to over seventy years in 1960.

For reasons that are not well understood, the reproductive life of a woman is growing longer at both ends. The average age at menarche (beginning of the menses) in the United States is thirteen instead of fourteen or fifteen a century ago, and many women who are fifty have not yet reached menopause. With this in mind let us examine the various factors that may, but need not, affect late motherhood.

Decreased Fertility

All other conditions being the same, the probability of conception decreases with increasing age. It is not well understood why this is so. It may be connected with the fact that, according to Dorothy Nortman of the Population Council, "unlike the female of almost all other species, the human female is unique in that the stock of oocytes [immature egg cells present at birth] is virtually exhausted early in life."

Dr. G. B. Talbert reported that by the ages of thirty-nine to forty-five the supply of oocytes in an ovary had dwindled to about 11,000, from a stock of about 250,000 present at birth. Most of the oocytes must thus have disintegrated, since a woman only matures 400 to 500 during her reproductive years.

In addition there is also considerable evidence from both human and animal studies that age affects the quality as well as the quantity of the oocytes. The quality of sperm may also deteriorate with age.

Since, as we discussed in Chapter 14, almost all imperfect zygotes and fetuses are aborted spontaneously, this may partially account for the considerable increase in abortions with parental age.

Increased Risk to the Mother

One has only to stroll through an old cemetery, even in a very young country like the United States, to realize that childbearing used to be extremely hazardous. If one examines the memorial brasses still found in English churches, one often sees the effigy of a husband flanked by three wives, one or two of whom may have died during childbirth.

During the nineteenth and twentieth centuries childbearing has become relatively safe. In 1974 maternal mortality rates for women in the Western world was under 35 per 100,000 live births.

The risk, however, increases with increase in maternal age. It is ten times as dangerous for a woman in her forties to have a baby as for one in her twenties. Let us stress once more that since the overall mortality is low, the risk is still relatively small.

Death during pregnancy and delivery can be due to causes specifically related to pregnancy, as well as to aggravation by the stresses and strains of pregnancy of unrelated conditions. Older women obviously have a higher risk of dying from such illnesses as heart disease than younger ones. But with good medical care the risk can be considerably reduced.

Most of the deaths directly due to pregnancy are caused by toxemia—a complication of pregnancy characterized by high blood pressure and sometimes even convulsions, hemorrhage, and infectious disease (sepsis). The incidence of these conditions, which may occur as complications of pregnancy, increases with age, though here again good medical care minimizes ill effects.

The incidence of toxemia in particular increases by a factor of 3 to 4 with the age of the mother.

There is also some truth to the commonly held belief that age has an adverse effect on delivery. Older mothers have more than their share of long labors, poorly dilating cervixes, malpresented fetuses (any position of the baby during birth except head first), and Caesarean sections. And older mothers have a higher incidence of postpartum hemorrhage caused by uterine inertia (insufficient uterine contractions) after delivery.

All these complications can normally be handled without too much difficulty at a modern, well-equipped medical center.

Increased Risk to the Fetus and Child

The greatest concern of older parents by far is the possibility that their baby will be abnormal.

The incidence of Down's Syndrome, the most common of

the congenital birth defects, rises considerably with increasing age. The increased occurrence of this birth defect is so striking that the age of the mother itself has been considered to be the cause, though mongoloid babies have been born to very young women.

A recent detailed study by Ernest B. Hook, of New York State's Birth Defects Institute, indicates that at the upper limit of the reproductive age the incidence of babies born with Down's Syndrome increases from year to year.

Whereas there is approximately 1 incidence of Down's Syndrome per 1,500 live births for women in their twenties, the rate increases to 1 in 527 women at age thirty-four; 1 in 413 for women aged thirty-five; 1 in 183 for women aged thirty-eight; and 1 in 83 for women aged 41.

There has been much speculation about the cause for this increase. It has been suggested that Down's Syndrome occurs more frequently when the egg of the woman has to "wait" in the Fallopian tube to be fertilized after it has been expelled from the ovary. This state of affairs, it is said, occurs more frequently in older women than their younger counterparts. This is, however, only one of several theories.

The increased incidence of Down's Syndrome might also be associated with the presumed general decline of the quality of the egg cells of the ovary.

It was always assumed that the extra chromosome attached to Pair 21 was contributed by the mother. It has recently been reported at the American Society of Human Genetics that the father, too, can contribute the extra twenty-first chromosome.

The increased incidence of birth defects in older women is independent of the number of children a woman has had. Thus, the third child of a woman aged thirty-five has as great or as small a chance of being born with a birth defect as the first child of a woman of the same age.

Today, through amniocentesis (see Chapter 18) the older child-bearing couple can be virtually certain whether or not their child will have Down's Syndrome. The disease is such a heavy burden both for the parents and society at large that a California legislator has attempted to introduce a bill into Congress that would require all mothers over thirty-five to undergo amniocentesis.

In addition to Down's Syndrome there are about 100 different chromosomal abnormalities compatible with survival of the baby. Most of these result from spontaneous mutations (changes) that can take place in the chromosome of either the mother or the father. In every living creature, including man, the incidence of these mutations increases with age. This is why older parents have a slightly greater proportion of children affected by these types of birth defects than younger parents. These birth defects are of so many different types, and fortunately so rare, that they are not identified on a routine amniocentesis.

Not every couple who is told that their child will be abnormal will opt for abortion. The decision is a very personal one, and depends to a large extent on the religious and ethical conviction of the patients. It is recommended that those who face this difficult decision discuss the matter with a suitably trained genetic counselor.

Psychological Impact

Sweet as they are, babies require a tremendous amount of attention. They sometimes exhaust the youngest parents and can be especially hard on older ones. Fortunately the time during which a child requires intensive care is relatively short. As one woman, who only became a mother when she was forty, put it: "The years pass quickly—it is the days that are so incredibly long."

Older parents do have their share of worries, including financial ones. College-age children often need financial help from their parents at a time when the latter have already passed the peak of their earning capacity. Many an older parent also feels that he or she may not be able to complete the job of raising a child. Here again the progress made by medicine should be a reassuring factor.

On the other hand parents report that having their children when they are less absorbed by their own growth adds another dimension of pleasure. Many couples, who by accident or design produce, as one mother put it, "their own grandchildren," report that a late addition to an already existing family is a great delight.

For the couple who has had to overcome an infertility problem, parenthood usually is especially rewarding. One young woman whose first child was not conceived for years said, "Each time they brought me my baby in the hospital I fell asleep. For years I had not felt as relaxed as I did when I saw Judy. To me she was the greatest thing in the world, next to God. I just felt that everybody should admire her. I knew that my attitude would perhaps make my baby feel too special, but I just could not help it.

"This is why I decided to try to have a second child as soon as I could manage it. Once my body had learned how, I conceived within a matter of months. My children are less than two years apart. My husband and I just adore our two girls, but two are enough. After all these years of trying, I now wear an IUD."

With reasonable precautions older couples can have healthy babies, with whom, as it says in all fairy tales, "they will live happily almost forever after."

One-child Sterility

Melanie and Robert were married somewhat late in life. She was twenty-nine, he thirty-six. They decided to have children right away. To everyone's great joy Cathy was born fifteen months later. She turned out to be particularly delightful and Papa and Mama wanted her to have company.

When Cathy was about two, birth control was discontinued and Melanie expected to become pregnant in a matter of a few months. Nature ruled otherwise. A year later Cathy was still without a prospective sibling.

One-child sterility, as this condition is called, falls into two categories. The first includes couples who were not very fertile to begin with, but who were lucky because they conceived quickly the first time around. The second category consists of those whose fertility changed after they gave birth to the first child. Like primary infertility, these changes may have occurred in either the husband or the wife.

This book has detailed the long and tedious steps often necessary to uncover the cause of infertility. Couples who are serious about enlarging their families will have to be investigated as if a pregnancy never had taken place.

The senior author recalls a couple who were the parents of a healthy boy and had trouble conceiving for the second time. During the initial interview the young mother remembered that she had had an appendectomy when she was six years old. Examination of the scar indicated that the wound had been infected, and a culdoscopic exploration revealed many stringlike adhesions about the tubes and ovaries. Time and age had caused these bands of tissue to shrink and distort the tubes.

The tubes proved to be open, but they functioned poorly. Tubal patency could perhaps be restored surgically, but couples who are fortunate enough to have one child often feel that it is unwise to resort to such a major operation whose outcome is still so uncertain.

In this particular couple the fertility of the father was a contributory problem. His semen count might have been borderline to begin with. Now at thirty-three it was in a very low fertility range, perhaps because he was overweight, drank, and smoked heavily.

Luck must have been on this couple's side the first time around. Now their combined low fertility made it unlikely that they would succeed a second time.

Age, even if it involves only a couple of years, may be an important factor in a woman's decreased fertility. Minor defects in ovulation, perhaps characterized by slightly irregular periods, may have become more pronounced. Pregnancy, labor, and delivery itself may have damaged the delicate architecture of the reproductive organs. A minor, low-grade pelvic infection that went unnoticed by both the doctor and the patient may have affected the Fallopian tubes.

One-child sterility can also be caused by the consequences of a Caesarean section.

Sometimes the couple forgets events that occurred after they had their first child, especially if the offspring were spaced years apart.

Modern methods of birth control are also associated with a slight increase in infertility. In a very few women the anovulatory state induced by "the pill" persists even after the medication has been discontinued. Resumption of ovulation usually occurs on its own, after a period of a few months. If not, it can usually be corrected through the administration of one of the new fertility drugs, like Pergonal or Clomid.

The IUD, again only in a very small fraction of those who use it, can cause a low-grade pelvic inflammation which could result in scarring of the Fallopian tubes. Such low-grade infections may also result from surgically induced abortions.

Finally, the increased incidence of venereal disease, among both men and women, is closely associated with the rise in VD-induced infertility.

Most couples have a difficult time accepting their infertility. The problem is usually more easily handled from an emotional point of view if there is already a child in the family.

Nobody knows the incidence of one-child sterility, because people are most reluctant to talk about their infertility, whether total or partial.

We all like to think that we are masters of our destiny. It is hard to admit in public that we really wanted a houseful of children when we only managed to produce one.

20

DESTERILIZATION

In surgery, eyes first and most; fingers next and little; tongue last and least.

—Sir George Murray Humphry

OVER 8 MILLION PERSONS IN THE UNITED STATES NOW RELY ON SURGICAL sterilization for birth control, and the number is steadily growing. Most of those who opt to end their fertility in such a permanent manner remain completely satisfied with their decision. Many report a freer, more uninhibited sex life, and most say that they are willing to abide by their decision no matter what happens to their marriage or children. A very few—one-half of 1 percent—change their minds and seek out physicians who are willing to attempt to undo the supposedly permanent. Not all those who gather information on the subject will actually undergo the operation.

According to a May 1976 survey published in *Population Reports*, the reasons given for these changes of heart fall into four categories. The first, and by far the most common, is remarriage after the divorce or death of the former spouse. The other three are: death of one or more children; improved economic situation; or the psychological desire to overcome the supposed ill effects of sterilization.

Whatever the reason, regaining fertility once it has been

given up is, according to a recent article in *Medical World News,* "A Tough Road to Travel."

In the male, sterilization (vasectomy) involves the severing of the two vasa deferentia, the foot-long connections between the epididymis and the seminal vesicle. In the woman, sterilization (tubal ligation) involves blocking a small portion of both Fallopian tubes. In women the initial approach is either abdominal or vaginal, with a specially equipped culdoscope or laparoscope.

At present the success rate of reversing voluntary sterilization is still rather low. Although figures vary from physician to physician, the most commonly heard estimate is about 25 percent. These figures are not very reliable since many factors (age, minor defects in a new partner of untested fertility) affect conception in various ways.

It is almost self-evident that the fertility of the other partner must be established before desterilization is attempted.

The surgical techniques utilized to undo either a vasectomy or a tubal ligation are the same as those employed to repair a defective vas deferens or a nonfunctional tube.

Vasectomy Reversal (Vasovasostomy)

Even though the man will eventually undergo the operation, urologists are almost unanimous in reporting that the first contact or inquiry about turning a vasectomy (known as vasovasostomy or vas anastomosis) is always made by the prospective mother.

It takes only about twenty minutes and anywhere from $65 to $250 to perform a vasectomy. Reversing the operation is a much more complicated, risky, and costly process. Whereas the original procedure is done under local anesthesia, and as an out patient, a reversal requires general anesthesia, takes about two hours, and usually requires a four-day stay in the hospital. In 1977 the operation and related costs tallied an average of $2,500, and, since medical costs seem to be constantly on the rise, the undertaking may become even more expensive.

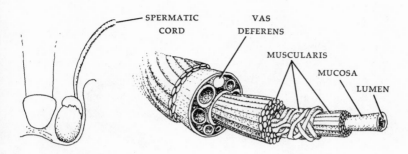

Even something as narrow as the vas deferens has many layers.

A lengthy procedure like a vasovasostomy always presents a certain operative risk. Complications include testicular hemorrhage, which very occasionally entails the loss of a testicle. Yet most urologists specializing in male infertility work report that they are able and willing to try to help their patients.

PROCEDURE

One of the great difficulties is that the vas deferens, which was cut during the original procedure (see drawing), is as thin as a wisp. From the outside the cross section measures a mere 1/8 inch, but the vas is not a simple hollow tube like an ordinary garden hose. The inner tract through which the sperm must travel is only a tiny slit, measuring approximately 1/25th inch in diameter. Like the Fallopian tubes the vas deferens is equipped with muscle and nerve tissue that facilitate sperm transport.

Techniques vary from surgeon to surgeon, but the one used most frequently goes approximately as follows. The physician first cuts into the scrotum enclosing the testicles, one of the toughest membranes of the body. Then the thin, spaghetti-like vas deferens is lifted out. The scarred stumps are located, and the segment of the vas leading back to the testicle (proximal vas end) is cut back until the surgeon notes that some thick, white gluelike material is protruding from the cut. This is the semen. The segment of the vas that leads to the seminal vesicle

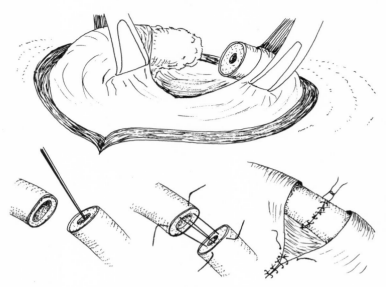

Commonly used procedure for the repair of the vas deferens

(distal vas end) is also neatly sliced off until all scar tissue has been removed.

To ensure that no obstruction remains, a small stick (probe) is gently inserted into the two open ends. Then the two cleaned stumps are brought together (this particular procedure is called an end-to-end anastomosis), and sewn with a needle as fine as an eyelash and very, very thin surgical suturing material. Some surgeons insert a small splint into the inner canal of the vas while it heals. Others feel that the complications that may accompany the removal of the splint offset whatever good its presence might have provided.

There is also some discussion among surgeons about whether it is best to suture the lining of the vas (the mucosa) together or only to suture the outside layer.

Though end-to-end anastomosis is by far the most common procedure, some physicians attempt to reunite a vas by suturing the two ends side to side and making a small opening between the tubes.

If the original cut was made near the epididymis—the long passage between the testicles and the vas itself—the surgeon may connect the severed end of the vas to the epididymis. So far the procedure has not been used very often.

No matter what procedure is opted for, the operation is so delicate that many surgeons now use microsurgery techniques.

Regardless of the procedure used, the postoperative care of the devasectomized patient is more or less standard. Patients are asked to wear a scrotal support for seven to fourteen days, and to abstain from sexual intercourse for ten to fourteen days. Some physicians supplement the surgery with drug therapy. Commonly prescribed drugs are: antibiotics, thyroid hormone and/or a cortisone-like compound. The latter two drugs are believed to stimulate spermatogenesis. The semen of the patient is analyzed after a period of three weeks and regularly thereafter for a period of one year.

There are very few before and after sperm counts, since most men who underwent a vasectomy in the first place did not have an infertility problem and hence had no use for a count. Nevertheless there is a general consensus that sperm counts decrease from prevasectomy levels. A single study made by Dr. H. Y. Lee on 178 patients indicates a drop of about 33 percent from prevasectomy levels. In data obtained in a vasectomy reversal experiment carried out by Dr. N. J. Alexander and his colleagues on Rhesus monkeys, the sperm count returned to prevasectomy levels after eight weeks, which is better than results obtained in men, perhaps because the time during which the monkeys were vasectomized was shorter.

At present there is no clear-cut evidence on whether any one of the above techniques is more successful than another. The end-to-end anastomosis technique is the only one that has been used widely. There is some indication that microsurgical techniques are somewhat more successful, but the number of cases reported so far is too small to be conclusive.

According to a survey published in *Population Reports,* there is surprisingly little follow-up among patients who underwent vasectomy reversal. In some studies only 50 percent of the patients bothered to report back to their surgeons. One author suggests that this may reflect indifference on the part of the patient, who may have felt pressure from a partner to restore his fertility and who feels he has done his part by undergoing the operation.

SUCCESS

The ultimate proof of desterilization is the achievement of pregnancy. Success of vasectomy reversal is, however, divided into two parts. The first is the "anatomical" success, defined as the appearance of normal sperm in the ejaculate; the second is the "functional" success, as determined by pregnancy.

About 50 percent of vasectomy reversals are anatomical successes. Among the complications that arise are the formation of small, benign tumors, sometimes caused by the leakage of sperm from the epididymis or the vas into the surrounding tissue, and inflammation that can result in adhesions and scar tissue formation.

After the original vasectomy the end of the vas connected to the testicle (proximal vas) has a tendency to enlarge, while the end connected to the epididymis does not. It sometimes may be difficult to align these two ends properly, thus failing to reestablish a suitable pathway for the sperm. Reversal of vasectomies done in the convoluted portion of the vas, and in patients in whom a large segment of the vas was removed, also usually give poor results. Other factors, such as injury to the nervous system during the original operation, or the repair, which can interfere with sperm transport and its deposition in the female tract, may also play a role.

SPERM ANTIBODIES

Unfortunately repairing the vas in such a way that viable sperm is again being ejaculated is only part of the battle. About 50 percent of men undergoing vasectomy develop antibodies to their own sperm (see Chapter 17) that interfere with the fertilization of the ovum. Combining the number of anatomical failures with those due to sperm antibodies, one comes up with a success rate of approximately 25 percent, which is not very encouraging. Progress is made in removing sperm antibodies by washing the sperm and then using it for homologous artificial insemination. Drugs to suppress sperm antibodies are also used on an experimental basis.

Nearly all patients who now wish to reverse their vasectomies say that they made the decision to have the operation after full and extensive counseling. Some of the patients who seek reversal do, after some more counseling, decide that such an attempt—even if successful—is not going to solve their present problem. It is, for instance, unrealistic to attempt to replace a child lost in a tragedy; and those partners who remarry after their first marriage broke up in spite of children, do understand that children per se do not ensure a successful marriage. They too may decide to forgo such a costly procedure. Some men, however, are willing to undergo more than one operation to restore their fertility.

Research is being done at present to develop semipermanent vasectomy methods. Clips and plugs that can be removed at will are being tried in various parts of the world, and the surgical techniques used in reversing the operation should improve.

The development of frozen sperm banks in which men can store some of their sperm before they undergo a vasectomy may become an insurance system for men who think that conceivably fate may cause them to change their mind.

Desterilization in Women

Physicians are not much more enthusiastic about reversing tubal ligation than they are about undoing vasectomies.

The operation itself is very similar to the one used to repair Fallopian tubes that have become obstructed as a consequence of some pelvic disease or trauma. It involves major abdominal surgery, which should never be undertaken lightly. As in the case of the male reversal, the ultimate success of the operation depends very much on the extent of the original surgery. An oviduct whose architecture was extensively destroyed by disease is much more difficult to fix than one blocked by a minor adhesion.

There is a great discrepancy in the reported success rates of female desterilization. Dr. Arthur Haskin of the University of Maryland reports a success rate of 80 percent in a group of fifteen to twenty women, whereas Dr. Robert Wheeless, Jr., of Johns Hopkins says 20 to 40 percent is the best result one can expect. Dr. Wayne Decker, of the New York Fertility Research Foundation, estimates a success rate of 10 to 50 percent, depending largely on the technique used to ligate the tubes initially. Tubes interrupted by burning with an electric current are most difficult to repair and so give the poorest results. Newer techniques using microscopic stitches offer encouragement for improved results.

Requests for the female reversal operation have so far remained at a rate below those for vasectomy reversals, primarily because until recently tubal ligations were done less frequently than vasectomies.

The Fallopian tube is very large as compared to the vas deferens, and women do not develop antibodies to sperm or ova as a consequence of tubal ligation; nevertheless those undergoing reversal face a very serious complication. Any type of tubal surgery, including the one presently under consideration, increases the possibility of ectopic pregnancy—a condition which can be truly life-threatening if it is not diagnosed in time.

Again, as for vasectomy the search for a better, more reversible form of tubal ligation is under way. A clip like a bobby pin that is slipped onto both tubes near the uterine end seems promising. A tubal ligation using a clip can be performed in about eight minutes. The method is unfortunately associated with a much higher failure rate than the standard procedure. The clip method, however, was reversible in the one patient who requested it.

In conclusion it must be said that desterilization is still a novel art with a history of many more failures than successes. Though each couple, no doubt, has excellent reasons to reconsider the previous decision by one of the partners, regaining one's fertility is an even tougher proposition than overcoming a routine infertility problem.

FIVE

QUESTIONS AND ANSWERS

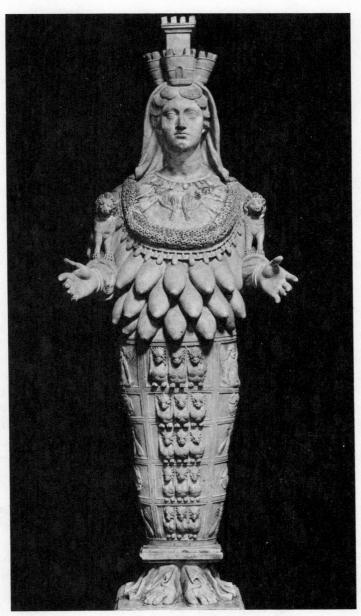

Diana of Ephesus, Goddess of Fertility (Courtesy of the Bettmann Archive)

21

FIFTY
FREQUENTLY
ASKED
QUESTIONS
ABOUT
INFERTILITY

1. *Does adoption improve fertility?*

This question is discussed so often that it almost seems to have become accepted as a fact that adoption improves fertility. Actually, when the problem was examined scientifically, it turned out not to be so. Most infertility patients who adopt a baby still continue with their treatment. There also is an element of chance in conception, and for some patients becoming pregnant takes very long. It might just happen after a baby has been adopted. This is especially true in cases where both partners are of borderline fertility.

2. *My temperature has gone up and my basal body temperature (BBT) chart indicates that I ovulated; why do I have to keep taking my temperature for the rest of the month?*

Your body temperature is a reflection of the hormones you produce. It increases with an increase in the progesterone level, decreases with the production of estrogen.

Each day from Day 1 to Day 28 in a normal menstrual cycle is important. Both phases of the cycle, the secretory (estrogen-dominated), and the luteal (progesterone-dominated) phase, must be normal to ensure proper preparation of the endometrium for implantation of the fertilized ovum.

Infertility and early abortion may result from improper preparation of the endometrium by progesterone. The condition can be identified by the failure of the temperature to rise after ovulation, or if after rising it does not stay elevated but gradually returns to the low level.

Though it is a bother, you must keep taking your temperature all the time throughout the menstrual cycle.

3. *When I wake up very early in the morning, should I take my temperature then even if I go back to sleep?*

No. Take your temperature at the usual time before you get out of bed.

4. *For how many days during each cycle is it possible for me to conceive?*

For three days. That is, two days before and the day of ovulation.

5. *What does the expression "biphasic" temperature mean?*

Normally your temperature stays up for two weeks and down for two weeks, i.e., there are two temperature phases. You can see the two plateaus quite easily when you look at the ideal BBT chart shown on page 76.

6. *Why do I menstruate (bleed) if I don't ovulate?*

The ovaries of patients who do not ovulate may still produce estrogen in a cyclical manner. This estrogen prepares the uterus for pregnancy. When the level of estrogen drops, you will bleed. Bleeding without ovulation is induced artificially in women who take the birth control pill, which indeed contains substances closely related to estrogen and progesterone. These women also do not ovulate, but bleed when the pill is withdrawn during the last seven days of an arbitrary menstrual cycle. This type of bleeding is called progesterone-withdrawal bleeding, or anovulatory bleeding.

7. *What happens to the egg if I don't become pregnant?*

Like the many superfluous sperm cells, it is disposed of by special white blood cells called phagocytes that operate as an efficient crew of sanitation workers, and digest matter no longer needed by the body.

8. *Do my ovaries take turns producing eggs each month?*

No. Your ovaries produce eggs in a random manner.

9. *I have only one ovary. Does this mean that I ovulate only every second month?*

No. Your one functioning ovary does double duty. It will produce an egg every month.

10. *I sometimes have pains in the pelvis during the middle of my cycle. Does this mean that I ovulate?*

This pain goes by the German name of *Mittelschmerz*—or "pain in the middle." It does not necessarily mean that you ovulate, though it can mean that. It may also mean that your ovaries swell and hurt without an egg being able to break out.

11. *Is clomiphene a hormone?*

No. Clomiphene is an anti-estrogen. It tricks the pituitary into producing more of its own ovulation-inducing hormone FSH. (See also Chapter 9 on Fertility Drugs.) Clomiphene is taken as a pill.

12. *Is Pergonal a hormone?*

Yes, Pergonal—the trade name for menotropins—is made up of the hormones FSH and LH. These natural hormones are produced abundantly by women during their menopause. They are recovered from the urine of these healthy women, refined, sterilized, and reduced to a powder. The powder is dissolved and given by injection. Both Clomid and Pergonal are powerful ovulation-inducers. Their administration must be closely supervised so that a woman does not produce too many ova at one time.

13. *What is human chorionic gonadotropin, and why do I have to take it together with Pergonal?*

Human chorionic gondadotropin is a special hormone initially made by the outer layer of the fertilized ovum—the chorion—and then by the placenta. It is given after therapy with Pergonal because it is believed to give the egg an extra push while it is being expelled from the ovarian follicle. HCG is the hormone in the urine of pregnant women that produces the positive pregnancy test.

14. *I only menstruate one or two days each month. Is that normal?*

A very scant or very long bleeding phase of the menstrual cycle may indicate some defect in the hormones responsible for menstruation.

15. *I sometimes stain slightly the day before I really start menstruating. Should I consider this Day 1 of my menstrual cycle?*

Yes you can, as long as you use the same system each month. If you are keeping a temperature chart, you may use the day when the temperature drops to the low level as Day 1.

16. *My breasts are very painful before I menstruate. Does this mean anything?*

During each menstrual cycle, and especially during pregnancy, the breasts are stimulated by hormones. This sometimes increases the blood flow to the breasts and may cause pain. Most women with painful breasts have no problem conceiving. In others it may indicate an excess production of estrogen, and hence some hormone abnormality.

17. *Why do I sometimes menstruate after intercourse?*

Such bleeding is definitely not related to menstruation and should be investigated very thoroughly. It might, for instance, be caused by a polyp, which in turn might interfere with conception.

18. *You asked whether my menstrual blood contains clots. Is that bad?*

It is not "bad" in the way this word is usually used, but the fact, if true, helps us diagnose your major problem. Clots may be caused by a fibroid, a polyp, or inflammation of the cervix (cervicitis), each of which may be the cause of your infertility.

19. *I only menstruate every 35 to 38 days. Will this affect my fertility?*

Some women regularly have very long cycles. The time between ovulation and the next menstrual cycle is very constant.

Delayed menstrual bleeding together with an erratic temperature chart may, however, result from failure to ovulate.

20. *Do fibroid tumors interfere with conception?*

Some women who have fibroids manage to conceive and sail through their pregnancy without any trouble. Others do have a major problem. The size of the tumor is not always a factor. A small fibroid located near the point of attachment of the Fallopian tubes may prevent conception, while a much larger one located elsewhere may not. The condition can now often be corrected by surgery. Since fibroids often are not responsible for infertility, *all* other factors that may contribute to the problem must be eliminated before surgery is undertaken. Fibroids, however, do have a tendency to grow. Large fibroids may interfere with the progress of pregnancy and labor. Women who are aware they have fibroids should have all the pregnancies they desire as soon as possible.

21. *What causes sperm antibodies?*

This is a complicated question that nobody quite yet has the answer to. What is known about these antibodies and how the condition is treated is discussed in Chapter 17 of this book.

22. *We have intercourse every day, sometimes twice. Why don't I become pregnant?*

It has been shown that couples who have intercourse frequently are more fertile than those who only copulate once a week, or two to three times a month. However, daily intercourse, when a couple is attempting to achieve pregnancy, may result in a decreased sperm count. For patients with an infertility problem we recommend some restraint before ovulation time, then intercourse two to three times during the fertile days of the woman. There is some evidence that long periods of abstinence may affect the motility and fertility potential of the sperm adversely.

23. *What causes a poor postcoital test?*

Low sperm count and diminished motility. Also the test may have been scheduled at the wrong time of the month.

Provided the sperm count of the man is normal, a poor postcoital test may be due to inhospitable cervical mucus in the woman. This can often be corrected rather easily with hormones. Sperm antibodies, which are more difficult to treat, may also be a factor (see Chapter 17).

24. *Does the amount of semen matter provided the count is normal?*

It can matter. The normal average volume of the ejaculate is 3 to 4 ml. Sperm that are contained in too large a volume (over 6ml. or a tablespoon) will have a low average number. If extreme, this can be corrected with homologous artificial insemination, using the husband's own sperm. It has been found that the first portion of the ejaculate contains most of the sperm. The physician may thus decide to use only this first portion for insemination. This is referred to as the split ejaculate technique.

If the sperm cells are too concentrated (total volume less than 1 ml.), many may perish in the vagina even before they make contact with the cervical mucus.

25. *After intercourse the semen runs right out of me. Does that keep me from becoming pregnant?*

Semen at the time of ejaculation is very viscous and sticky. Normally it becomes liquid in a few minutes. Sperm leave the seminal fluid and enter the cervical mucus in a very short time after intercourse. Women who want to conceive are advised to stay in bed, with their hips elevated by a pillow for fifteen minutes after intercourse.

26. *My sperm count seems to be different each time it is calculated. How low can it be for me still to impregnate my wife?*

Sperm counts often vary from ejaculate to ejaculate. This is no cause for concern as long as the count remains within normal limits. Pooling sperm for homologous artificial insemination sometimes helps those men who have a poor count but occasionally produce a good sample. (See Normal Count.)

27. *How should the semen be kept on its trip to the laboratory?*

It should be kept cool, below body temperature. After all, nature put the testicles outside the human body to ensure that the sperm is not overheated. Don't forget to stopper the tube, put the container in a paper bag, and carry it in your hand. Don't carry the specimen under your arm, and please keep it away from the car radiator.

28. *How soon after intercourse should the postcoital test be done?*

One to four hours is best.

29. *How often should we have intercourse?*

Two to three times a week is a good average figure for maximum fertility. However, your particular problem may be such that your physician suggests a different schedule.

30. *I took birth control pills for many years. Could they be responsible for my problem?*

They may. Birth control pills, which work by cutting out ovulation, have been shown to cause post-pill amenorrhea in some women. A normal menstrual cycle usually returns of its own accord after the pills have been discontinued for a number of months. Clomid—the anti-estrogen agent that indirectly stimulates the production of the gonadotropins by the pituitary

—has been used successfully to restore fertility. You might, of course, have had an infertility problem without knowing it before taking the pill, in which case it was totally unrelated to the birth control pills.

The pill may be especially injurious to women with a preexisting history of abnormal menstrual bleeding. Most women who have taken birth control pills conceive without trouble after discontinuing their use.

31. *I have been using an IUD for a number of years. Could it have affected my fertility?*

IUDs can cause pelvic inflammatory disease, which in turn can cause tubal defects that may result in infertility. The device may also cause scarring of the uterus. Though these things happen very rarely, the use of IUDs should be reserved for women who most likely are through with childbearing.

32. *I have been using a diaphragm for birth control. Could it have affected my fertility?*

Definitely not. An older name for the diaphragm is "Dutch cap," and it is just that—a "hat" for your cervix. Wearing it could not possibly affect your future fertility. Unfortunately many women have used a diaphragm for years only to find out later that one or both partners were infertile or even sterile.

33. *How can I tell whether I am immune to rubella?*

The body fights off all infections by making very specific antibodies. Some of these antibodies stay behind after the disease is over and can then be identified by a blood test.

Every woman should be certain of her rubella-immune status. Unless recently immunized, women should have such a test before they attempt to become pregnant. If the test is negative, it means that you have no rubella antibodies and should be vaccinated. Rubella vaccination can be as damaging to the fetus as the disease itself. Women who have been given a rubella vaccine should not become pregnant for four months following vaccination.

34. *What are adhesions?*

Injury or infectious disease may cause tissues to become inflamed. When two adjoining surfaces become inflamed, they often stick together. The healed tissue may remain fused.

Sometimes they pull apart except for some stringy, dense bands, which are called adhesions. If such adhesions form inside the narrow Fallopian tubes, they may effectively block the passage of sperm and egg. Adhesions can also form on the outside of the tubes and ovaries and interfere with conception. Adhesions often can be removed by surgery.

35. *Is endometriosis inherited?*

Not exactly, but it often runs in families.

36. *Does tubal surgery increase the chances of having a tubal pregnancy?*

Unfortunately, yes; however, your chances of becoming pregnant will have increased through surgery and your physician will watch you very carefully in order to avoid complications.

37. *Does endometriosis ever turn into cancer?*

At this moment your endometriosis is what may keep you from becoming pregnant. Endometrial growth very, very rarely becomes cancerous. Nevertheless all women should be checked regularly for cancer, especially if they have any cervical or uterine disorders, including endometriosis.

38. *I am very hairy. Does this have anything to do with my infertility problem?*

Perhaps. Excess body hair can simply be a family trait. Some women seem to be particularly sensitive to the male sex hormone, testosterone, that all women produce. They respond with superfluous hair growth on their faces, arms, and some-times chests. In some women hirsutism is caused by a true malfunction of the ovaries or the adrenals. These patients often have a male-type body hair distribution as well as defects in ovulation.

39. *Should I take thyroid pills?*

Only if your blood test reveals that your thyroid is slug-gish. Thyroid dysfunction plays a lesser role in infertility than was once assumed.

40. *What about vitamin pills, especially vitamin E?*

Most people who have a well-balanced diet do not need any extra vitamins except when their body undergoes extra stress as it does during pregnancy. Vitamin E has been endowed with all sorts of magical powers, including the prevention of aging and increased libido. As far as we know, none of these things are true. No scientist so far has been able to demonstrate a vitamin E deficiency in human beings. Unless your doctor tells you otherwise, no harm can come from taking a modest amount of multi-vitamin pills.

41. *What about all the other medications I am taking?*

An unborn child, especially early in pregnancy, seems to be particularly sensitive to the ill effects of medication. Medica-tion may also change the results of the delicate laboratory tests that you are undergoing. This is why it is important that you give a complete list of all the drugs you are taking to your doctor. This includes over-the-counter agents like aspirin, Ex-Lax, and vitamins. Let him or her be the judge of what you should or should not be taking.

42. *My doctor tells me that I should be tested for Barr bodies. What does this mean?*

When seen under the microscope all the cells obtained

from normal women have small dark specks, called Barr bodies after the scientist who discovered them. Barr bodies are useful for the diagnosis of Turner's Syndrome (see Chapter 18).

43. *My infertility problem makes me feel very isolated from my friends, who seem to have no troubles having children. Any suggestions?*

Most patients who have a serious medical problem feel very, very lonely. An infertility problem can cause great stress in a marriage.

Talking to other people who have a similar problem, or better still to a psychiatric social worker accustomed to helping patients with an infertility problem, relieves the loneliness. Unfortunately there are very few social workers so trained. Your gynecologist or infertility specialist may be able to help you identify a suitable therapist.

Speaking with other patients also helps. Some patients have gotten together simply by talking to each other in the doctor's waiting room. In any case it is good to realize that your problem cannot be that unique since it affects 10 to 15 percent of all marriages.

44. *I had my first child without any problems. Why do I have a problem now?*

For some women becoming pregnant is like playing roulette. You, as a couple, may have a low fertility, but you just happened to hit the jackpot the first time around. Some of the infertility problems discussed in this book may also develop with time. You may have had a minor infection, used birth control pills, developed a fibroid, a tumor, endometriosis. (See Chapter 19 which discusses one-child sterility.)

45. *Can one testicle produce enough sperm to impregnate?*

Yes, it definitely can.

46. *Can measles or mumps make a man sterile?*

These infectious diseases very rarely spread to the testicles, causing orchitis or inflammation of the testicles. Orchitis can, but need not, cause infertility. Orchitis usually only occurs when the patient develops these childhood diseases after puberty. Orchitis also hurts. So if you had mumps or measles, and do not remember your testicles being very painful at the time, you need not worry.

47. *What is a sperm count and how is it done?*

A sperm count is a test very much like a blood count, except that it is done on the ejaculate, that is used to determine the fertility status of the man. More details are given in Chapter 4.

48. *What are the causes of low sperm count?*

There are many different causes, such as a defect in the complex maturation process of the sperm. Sometimes a low sperm count results from the fact that the testicles remained undescended beyond the age of five years.

49. *What is a sperm bank?*

A place where sperm are frozen and stored to be used for artificial insemination. Most sperm banks contain donor sperm to be used when the male partner is infertile. There is a movement afoot to create sperm banks for men who opted for sterilization but want to keep some of their sperm "in the bank" in case they change their mind. So far nobody yet knows how many years frozen sperm will remain healthy and active.

50. *Do abnormal sperm cells mean that I will produce an abnormal fetus?*

No. Each ejaculate contains so many sperm cells that some are always abnormally shaped. These usually do not manage to fertilize the ovum.

GLOSSARY

ABORTION. Expulsion of a fetus during the first three months of pregnancy. It may be spontaneous or induced.

ACROSOME. Head of the sperm.

ADRENAL HYPERPLASIA. Overdevelopment of the adrenal gland accompanied by excess hormone production.

AID. See ARTIFICIAL INSEMINATION, DONOR SPERM.

AIH. See ARTIFICIAL INSEMINATION, HOMOLOGOUS.

AMNIOCENTESIS. Removal of a small amount of amniotic fluid by means of a syringe during the 14th to 16th week of pregnancy for diagnostic purposes (chromosome analysis).

ANEMIA. Too little oxygen-carrying protein (hemoglobin) in the blood or too few red blood cells.

ANTIBODY. Part of body's immunological response to "foreign" protein, including viruses, bacteria, and occasionally sperm cells.

APOCRINE GLANDS. Scent-producing glands.

ARTIFICIAL INSEMINATION, DONOR SPERM (AID). Insemination with sperm provided by a donor.

ARTIFICIAL INSEMINATION, HOMOLOGOUS (AIH). Insemination with the husband's sperm.

AZOSPERMIA. Absence of live sperm.

BARR BODY. Raw genetic material found in all cells of normal females but not in males.

BASAL BODY TEMPERATURE or BBT. Temperature taken in the morning before getting out of bed after a night of restful sleep.

BIOPSY. Surgical removal of tissue for purposes of diagnosis.

CANNULA. Small, hollow instrument used to introduce material into or remove it from the body cavity.

CAPACITATION. Processes in the female genital tract through which sperm become able to fertilize the ovum.

CERVICAL POLYPS. See POLYPS.

CERVICITIS. Inflammation of the cervix.

CERVIX. Neck of the uterus.

CHROMOSOMES. Thread-like arrangements of DNA in nucleus of the cell. They become visible only when the cell divides. Each human cell contains 46 chromosomes arranged in 23 pairs.

CLITORIS. Small, cylindrical structure of erectile tissue located above the opening of the urethra in the woman.

CLOMIPHENE CITRATE. A fertility pill. Also called Clomid.

CORPUS CAVERNOSUM. One of the cylinders making up the penis.

CORPUS LUTEUM. Temporary hormone production "plant" that develops in the ovarian follicle after the ovum is ejected. The corpus luteum secretes progesterone.

CORPUS SPONGIOSUM. One of the cylinders making up the penis.

CRYPTORCHISM. Undescended testicles.

CULDOSCOPY. Examination of the female pelvis with a culdoscope, a telescopic instrument inserted into the pelvis through the vagina.

DECKER CULDOSCOPE. Instrument developed by Dr. Albert Decker for the examination of the reproductive organs of a woman.

DESTERILIZATION. Reversing either vasectomy or tubal ligation.

DILATATION and CURETTAGE or (D & C). An operation during which the cervical canal is dilated and the uterine cavity is scraped with small, spoon-shaped instrument called a curette.

DNA. Short for deoxyribonucleic acid. The

nucleic acid "blueprint"
essential for transmission of
genetic information and
protein synthesis.

DOWN'S SYNDROME (also
called MONGOLISM or
TRISOMY 21). Birth defect
characterized by an extra
chromosome in chromosome
pair number 21.

ECTOPIC PREGNANCY.
Pregnancy outside the uterus.

ENDOMETRIAL BIOPSY.
Removal of a small amount
of the endometrium which is
examined under the
microscope to detect
abnormalities. See also
BIOPSY and
ENDOMETRIUM.

ENDOMETRIOSIS. Disease
characterized by the growth
of endometrial tissue outside
the uterus.

ENDOMETRIUM. Lining of the
uterus.

EPIDIDYMIS. Long, convoluted
duct conveying sperm from
the seminiferous tubules to
the vas deferens.

ESTROGEN. Major female sex
hormone.

FSH. See FOLLICLE
STIMULATING HORMONE.

FALLOPIAN TUBES. The long
funnel-shaped tubes on each
side of the uterus leading
from the ovaries to the uterus
that transport ova.
Fertilization takes place in the

Fallopian tubes. Also called
oviducts.

FERTILIZATION. Penetration
of ovum by sperm.

FIBROIDS. Benign tumors of
the uterus, also called leiomas
and myomas.

FIMBRIA. Fringes that form the
ends of the Fallopian tubes
and participate in the capture
of the ovum when it is
expelled from the ovary.

FOLLICLE. Small saclike
structure in which the ovum
matures.

FOLLICLE STIMULATING
HORMONE. This hormone,
emitted by the pituitary
gland, is identical in men and
women. At puberty it
promotes sexual maturation.
In the woman FSH is emitted
cyclically and initiates the
maturation of the primitive
egg cell in its special little
follicle—hence its name. In
men the hormone is essential
for sperm cell formation and
maturation.

FORESKIN. See PREPUCE.

FRUCTOSE. Type of sugar
essential for the normal
activity of sperm.

GENE. Biological unit of
heredity located in a definite
position on a particular
chromosome.

GONADOTROPIC
HORMONES. Hormones
formed in the pituitary that

affect the activity of the
ovaries or testes.

GONADS. Primary sex glands.
The ovaries in women and
the testes in men.

GONORRHEA. A widespread
venereal disease caused by a
bacterium called *Gonococcus
neisseria.*

HCG. See HUMAN
CHORIONIC
GONADOTROPIC
HORMONE.

HIRSUTISM. Hairiness.

HORMONES. Chemical
substances produced by
endocrine glands. Hormones
regulate various body
processes and metabolic
pathways.

HOSTILE MUCUS. Mucus that
immobilizes or destroys
sperm.

HUMAN CHORIONIC
GONADOTROPIC
HORMONE. Hormone
produced by the placenta
during pregnancy. Its
detection is the basis of
pregnancy tests.

HYDROCELE. Accumulation of
fluid around the testicle in
the scrotal sac.

HYDROTUBATION. Test that
uses fluid to determine
whether the Fallopian tubes
are unobstructed. The
procedure is also used as a
treatment of some tubal
defects.

HYMEN. Thin membrane
partially closing off the
vagina which ruptures upon
intercourse.

HYPOTHALAMUS. Gland in
the brain that is intimately
associated with the pituitary
in the control of ovulation
and other major body
functions.

HYSTERO-. Belonging or
referring to the uterus
(womb).

HYSTEROSALPINGOGRAM.
Picture of the uterus and
Fallopian tubes obtained by a
special X-ray technique.

IMPLANTATION. Process
during which a fertilized
ovum attaches itself to the
wall of the uterus.

IMPOTENCE. Inability to attain
or maintain erection.

INCOMPETENT CERVIX.
Premature dilation of the
cervix during pregnancy,
often resulting in miscarriage
or premature birth.

IUD (Intrauterine device): Small,
coillike object introduced into
the uterus for contraceptive
purposes.

KARYOTYPE. Photograph of
an arrangement of stained
chromosomes in pairs
according to size.

KLINEFELTER SYNDROME.
Genetic defect in males
characterized by an extra X
chromosome in the sex

chromosome pair. This results in atrophy of the testicles and sterility.

LH. See LUTEINIZING HORMONE.

LAPAROSCOPE. Diagnostic telescopic instrument used to examine the pelvic cavity.

LAPAROSCOPY. Examination of the abdominal and pelvic cavity with a laparoscope inserted through a small incision into the abdominal cavity.

LUTEAL PHASE. See SECRETORY PHASE.

LUTEINIZING HORMONE. This hormone, emitted by the pituitary gland, is identical in men and women. At puberty it promotes sexual maturation. In women LH is emitted cyclically and initiates the formation of the special temporary hormone production plant—the corpus luteum—which manufactures progesterone. In men the hormone, which also goes by the name of Interstitial Cell Stimulating Hormone, or ICSH for short, stimulates the development of the cells in the testicles that produce the male hormone testosterone.

MENARCHE. Time of life at which menses (menstruation) start.

MENOPAUSE. Time of life at which menses (menstruation) stop.

MISCARRIAGE. Expulsion of a fetus between the fourth and sixth month of pregnancy.

MITTELSCHMERZ. Abdominal pain some women experience at the time of ovulation.

MONGOLISM. See DOWN'S SYNDROME.

MORPHOLOGY. Structure or form.

MOTILITY. Ability (of sperm) to move.

MUCUS. Clear secretion from the mucous glands of any mucous membrane.

MYCOPLASM. Small, infectious microorganisms.

MYOMA. Benign growth (tumor) of the muscle tissue of the uterus.

NIDATION. Implantation— attachment of the fertilized ovum to the endometrium.

OLIGOMENORRHEA. Too infrequent menstruation.

OLIGOSPERMIA. Low sperm count.

OOCYTE. Primitive egg cell from which the ovum will develop.

ORCHITIS. Inflammation of the testicles.

OVARY. Primary sex organ of a woman.

OVIDUCTS. See FALLOPIAN TUBES.

OVULATION. Escape of the ovum from the ovary.

PAP SMEAR (short for Papanicolaou smear). Process during which a few cells are removed from cervical canal and examined under the microscope. Commonly used to detect early cancer of the uterine cervix.

PERGONAL. A fertility medication; the hormone FSH extracted from the urine of postmenopausal women. It is used to induce ovulation.

PITUITARY GLAND. Small gland located at the base of the brain manufacturing many hormones including FSH and LH.

POLYCYSTIC OVARIES. Disease characterized by ovaries studded with follicle cysts, which are unerupted, partially developed ova. Also termed Stein-Leventhal disease.

POLYP. A small, usually benign growth on a stalk that can occur, among other places, in the uterus or cervix.

POSTCOITAL TEST. Examination of cervical mucus shortly after intercourse to discover whether cervical mucus and sperm are compatible.

PREPUCE. The skin covering the head of the penis. It is often removed in the newborn infant by circumcision. Also called foreskin.

PROGESTERONE. Major female sex hormone, called the "hormone of pregnancy."

PROLIFERATIVE PHASE. Portion of the menstrual cycle (following menstruation until after ovulation) dominated by estrogen.

PROSTATE GLAND. A gland encircling the male urethra that manufactures some of the fluid making up the ejaculate.

PROSTATITIS. Inflammation of the prostate.

RETARDATE EJACULATION. Ejaculation that takes place after withdrawal of the penis from the vagina. In some men this may become an involuntary reflex.

RETROGRADE EJACULATION. During ejaculation sperm is deposited in the bladder instead of exiting through the urethra.

RUBIN TEST. Test developed by Dr. Isidore Rubin in which gas is introduced through the Fallopian tubes under pressure to determine whether they are open.

SALPINGO-. Referring to the Fallopian tubes.

SALPINGOGRAM. X-ray picture of the Fallopian tubes.

SALPINGOLYSIS. Removal of

small adhesions around the Fallopian tubes.

SALPINGOPLASTY. Repair of the Fallopian tubes by surgical methods.

SCROTUM. Tough skin sac enclosing the testicles.

SECRETORY PHASE. Portion of the menstrual cycle (that lasts for the 14 days following ovulation) dominated by progesterone. Also called the luteal phase.

SEMINAL VESICLE. Outbudding at the upper end of the vas deferens manufacturing fructose and other nutrients essential for sperm capacitation.

SEMINIFEROUS. Seed-carrying.

SPECULUM. (Vaginal.) Instrument for opening the vagina to permit direct inspection.

SPERM COUNT. Test to determine the number and nature of sperm produced by an individual male.

SPERMATOZOON. Fully developed male sex cell (plural is spermatozoa).

SPINNBARKEIT. Term used to describe the consistency of cervical mucus.

STEIN-LEVENTHAL OVARIES. See POLYCYSTIC OVARIES.

TESTOSTERONE. Principal male sex hormone.

TURNER'S SYNDROME. A genetic defect in females characterized by congenital failure of the ovaries to develop and abnormal bone development.

UTERINE POLYPS. See POLYPS.

UTERUS. Also called womb. The pear-shaped, hollow organ of reproduction in which the fertilized ovum implants and the baby develops during pregnancy.

VAGINA. Genital canal of a woman, extending outward from uterus.

VAGINISMUS. Involuntary, strong contractions of the vagina when intercourse is attempted.

VARICOCELE. Varicose veins in the scrotal sac.

VAS DEFERENS. Duct connecting the epididymis to the urethra.

VASECTOMY. Surgical severance of the vas deferens, usually undergone voluntarily to achieve sterility.

VENEREAL DISEASE. Infection transmitted primarily during intercourse.

INDEX

Index

antibiotics, effects of, 114, 116
antibodies, 39, 71, 179–183,
210–211, 222, 225
anti-estrogen, 98, 220
appendicitis, infection from, 117
aprocine glands, 57–58
artificial insemination, 168–178;
drug therapy with, 99; history
of, 169; legitimacy and, 170;
secrecy of, 169–170, 177;
sperm bank for, 171–172,
229; timing of, 80
artificial insemination, donor
sperm (AID): definition of,
168; donor selection for,
175–176; for homosexual
couples, 174; results of,
177–178; sexual love and,
173; for single women, 174;
technique of, 176–177; uses
of, 173–174
artificial insemination,
homologous (AIH): definition
of, 168; uses of, 167,
171–173, 223
aspermia, 38
aspirin, effects of, 227
astenozoospermia, 38
autosomal chromosomes,
187–188, 193
azospermia, 38, 39, 41

Babasco plant, 151
"Band-Aid" surgery, 88
Baramki, Theodore A., 129
Barr, M. L., 193–194
Barr body, 193–194, 227–228
basal body temperature (BBT):
chart for, 73–80, 218–219,
221; definition of, 74;
variations in 78–79, 222
belly-button surgery, 88
Biddeman, Miriam, 13–22
biological clock, 57

biopsy: definition of, 46;
endometrial, 71–73; testicular,
41, 45
biphasic temperature, 219
birth control: BBT and, 80;
progesterone and, 151;
surgical sterilization for,
205–206
birth control pill: effects of, 99,
112–113, 151–152, 204,
224–225; invention of, 95,
98; as treatment for ovarian
failure, 111
birth defects, 184–195; age as
factor in, 199–201;
clomiphene therapy and, 101;
percentage of, 186
Birth Defects Institute, 200
bladder, semen in, 48–49
blastocyst, 148
Boston Hospital for Women, 22
Bozzoni, Philip, 87
breast pain, 221
breast secretion, 105–106
Bromerzocryptin, 105

Caesar, Julius, 127
Caesarian section: age as factor
in, 199; effects of, 204;
naming of, 127; use of, 127,
150
cancer, 65–66, 226
canker sore, 58
cannula, 83
capacitation, 30–31
Carnegie Institute of
Embryology, 145
carriers of genetic diseases, 193
Celsus, 95
cerclage, 128, 149
cervical canal, 30, 55, 67–69
cervical cancer, 65–66
cervical mucus test, 67–69
cervical os, 55

immune factors, *see* antibodies
implantation, defects in,
147–149
impotence, 15, 38, 39, 41,
163–165
incompetent cervix, 128,
149–150
infections, 82, 114–120
infectious diseases, 47, 65–66,
69, 82, 93–94
infertility: causes of, 8–9 (table);
counseling for, 12–22;
diagnosis of, 35–42 (male),
63–94 (female); prevalence of,
3, 238; psychological
adjustment to, 19–22;
treatment of, 43–49 (male),
95–153 (female); VD and,
204
infertility evaluation: resistance
to, 36; time required for, 63
Ingersoll, F. M., 131
insulin, 32
intercourse: frequency of, 8–9,
157–158, 161, 222–223, 224;
pain during, 161; timing of,
79, 195
intrauterine devices (IUD),
effects of, 117, 204, 225
iodine, as thyroid test, 45
isolation, infertility and, 228

Johansen, Karl Eric, 47
Johns Hopkins, 129, 212
Johnson, Virginia E., 162
Jones, Howard W., 129
Josephine, Empress, 64

karyotype, 187–190
Kennedy family, 185
Khatamee, Masood A., 120
Kistner, Robert W., 98
Kleegman, Sophie, 169
Klinefelter Syndrome, 188, 194

labia, 53
labor, age as factor in, 199
laparascope, 88, 90–91
laparoscopy, 82–83, 87–94
laparotomy, 88
Larson, G. Douglas, 125
Ledger, William J., 114–115
Lee, H. Y., 209
Leeuwenhoek, Anton van,
25–26, 35
leioma, *see* fibroid tumor
lesions, 46–47
LH, *see* luteinizing hormone
Lieber, Ernest, 191
Long Island Jewish Hospital,
191
lovemaking, fertility and, 4
luteal phase, 61, 218–219
luteinizing hormone (LH), 33,
43–44, 58–61, 97–98,
101–102, 103

male organs of reproduction,
25–34
male sexual dysfunction,
163–167
Malone, L. J., 131
mandrake plant, 95
Mann, Edward C., 144–145
marital maladjustment, 6,
157–167
Marker, Russell, 151
Massachusetts General Hospital,
131
Masters, William H., 162
masturbation, 14, 35, 36, 166
maternal mortality rates,
198–199
measles, effects of, 228–229
Medical World News, 206
medication, side effects of, 49,
78, 227
meiosis, 186–187
menarche, 126, 197–198

Index

ovary, single, 220
overpopulation problem, 19, 30
oviducts, see Fallopian tubes
ovulation: BBT and, 73, 79;
failure of, 70, 96–97, 222;
hormones and, 57–62, 71,
101–106, 220; menstrual
cycle and, 61, 64, 66, 67–69,
219; test for, 71–73
ovum (egg): function of, 25, 31,
221; production and discharge
of, see ovulation; relative size
of, 30. See also oocyte

palpating, 65–66
pap smear, 65–66
Paracelsus Clinic for Barren
Couples (Frankfurt,
Germany), 132
patency, determination of, 82
pathologist, definition of, 46
pelvis: examination of, 65–66,
87–91; inflammation in, 82,
116, 117, 225; pain in, 58,
220
penicillin, 114, 116
penis, 26–27, 54
Penthouse Forum, 163–164
Pergonal, 101–105, 204,
220–221
peritoneal cavity, 83, 87–91
phagocytes, 220
phenylketonuria, 190
phocomelia, 146
p.i.d. (pelvic inflammatory
disease), 116, 225
pituitary gland: disorders of,
43–44, 105, 109; feedback
mechanism of, 97–99;
function of, 33, 43–44, 45,
58–61, 67–69, 220; in
menopause, 102; tumor, 105
placenta, 148, 150, 221
Planned Parenthood, 22

polycistic (Stein-Leventhal)
ovaries, 98, 99, 101, 109–112
polyp, 128, 221, 222
polyspermia, 38
Population Council, 198
population explosion, 19, 30
Population Reports, 205
postcoital test, 36, 70–71, 223,
224
postpartum hemorrhage, 199
post-pill amenorrhea, 99,
112–113
Pratt, Joseph, 12–13
pregnancy: attitudes toward, 16,
17; death during, 199;
ectopic, 138–140, 147, 212;
motivation for, 6–7;
progesterone and, 61, 98
pregnanediol, 150–151
prepuce, 26
progesterone: BBT and, 73, 218;
feedback mechanism of,
97–98; function of, 67, 150;
pregnancy and, 61, 98;
production of, 33, 60, 61,
151; test for, 71–80;
treatment with, 150–152;
withdrawal of, 111, 219
progestins, synthetic, 151–152
prolactic hormone, 105–106
proliferative phase, 60
prostate gland, 30
prostatitis, 9
pseudopregnancy, 124

rectum, 57, 66
Recurrent Miscarriage Clinic of
New York Hospital, 144–145
replacement therapy, 43
reproductive organs, 25–34,
53–62
Resolve, Inc., 22
retardate ejaculation, 163–167
retrograde ejaculation, 48–49